NURSING PHOTOBOOK™

# Giving
# Medications

*NURSING81* BOOKS
INTERMED COMMUNICATIONS, INC.
HORSHAM, PENNSYLVANIA

## NURSING81 BOOKS

### NURSING PHOTOBOOK™ SERIES
Providing Respiratory Care
Managing I.V. Therapy
Dealing with Emergencies
Giving Medications
Assessing Your Patients
Using Monitors
Providing Early Mobility
Giving Cardiac Care
Performing GI Procedures
Implementing Urologic Procedures
Controlling Infection
Ensuring Intensive Care
Coping with Neurologic Disorders
Caring for Surgical Patients
Working with Orthopedic Patients
Nursing Pediatric Patients
Helping Geriatric Patients
Attending Ob/Gyn Patients
Aiding Ambulatory Patients
Carrying Out Special Procedures

### NURSING SKILLBOOK® SERIES
Reading EKGs Correctly
Dealing with Death and Dying
Managing Diabetics Properly
Assessing Vital Functions Accurately
Helping Cancer Patients Effectively
Giving Cardiovascular Drugs Safely
Giving Emergency Care Competently
Monitoring Fluid and Electrolytes Precisely
Documenting Patient Care Responsibly
Combatting Cardiovascular Diseases Skillfully
Coping with Neurologic Problems Proficiently
Using Crisis Intervention Wisely
Nursing Critically Ill Patients Confidently

### NURSE'S REFERENCE LIBRARY™
Diseases

### Nursing81 DRUG HANDBOOK™

**NURSING PHOTOBOOK™ Series**

PUBLISHER
Eugene W. Jackson

EDITORIAL DIRECTOR
Jean Robinson

CLINICAL DIRECTOR
Barbara McVan, RN

ART DIRECTOR
Lisa A. Gilde

**Intermed Communications
Book Division**

DIRECTOR
Daniel L. Cheney

RESEARCH DIRECTOR
Elizabeth O'Brien

PRODUCTION AND PURCHASING DIRECTOR
Bacil Guiley

**Staff for this volume**

BOOK EDITOR
Richard Samuel West

CLINICAL EDITOR
Helene Ritting Nawrocki, RN

ASSOCIATE EDITOR
Katherine W. Carey

PHOTOGRAPHER
Paul A. Cohen

DESIGNER
Linda Jovinelly Franklin

CLINICAL EDITORIAL ASSOCIATE
Mary Gyetvan, RN, BSEd

EDITORIAL/GRAPHIC COORDINATOR
Doreen K. Stowers

COPY EDITOR
Barbara Hodgson

EDITORIAL ASSISTANT
Evelyn M. James

PHOTOGRAPHY ASSISTANT
Thomas Staudenmayer

DESIGN ASSISTANTS
Lorraine Lostracco Carbo
Darcy Moore Feralio

DARKROOM ASSISTANT
Gary Donnelly

ART PRODUCTION MANAGER
Wilbur D. Davidson

ART ASSISTANTS
Diane Fox            Sandra Simms
Robert Perry         Louise Stamper
Robert H. Renn       Ron Yablon

RESEARCHER
Vonda Heller

TYPOGRAPHY MANAGER
David C. Kosten

TYPOGRAPHY ASSISTANTS
Ethel Halle
Diane Paluba

PRODUCTION MANAGER
Robert L. Dean, Jr.

PRODUCTION ASSISTANT
M. Eileen Hunsicker

ILLUSTRATORS
Jean Gardner         John R. Murphy
Tom Herbert          Robert Smith
Robert Jackson       Bud Yingling
Cynthia Mason

SERIES GRAPHIC DESIGNER
John C. Isely

COVER PHOTO
Seymour Mednick

**Clinical consultants
for this volume**
Nancy Burns, RN, MS
Assistant Professor of Nursing
Director of Continuing Education
University of Texas at Arlington
School of Nursing
Arlington, Texas

Lenora Haston, RN, BSN
Former Clinical Coordinator for Surgery
Temple University Hospital
Philadelphia, Pennsylvania

Copyright © 1981, 1980 by Intermed
Communications, Inc.,
132 Welsh Road, Horsham, PA 19044
All rights reserved. Reproduction in
whole or part by any means
whatsoever without written permission
of the publisher is prohibited by law.
Printed in the United States of America.

030681

Library of Congress Cataloging in Publication Data

Main entry under title:
Giving medications

(Nursing Photobook)
Bibliography: p.
Includes index.
1. Drugs Administration    II. Nursing
RM147.G58      615'6      80-14474
ISBN 0-916730-22-0

# Contents

Introduction

## Beginning the procedure

CONTRIBUTORS TO
THIS SECTION INCLUDE:
Helene Ritting Nawrocki, RN
Minnie Rose, RN, BSN, MEd

**8** Preparations and precautions

## Administering by the gastrointestinal route

CONTRIBUTORS TO
THIS SECTION INCLUDE:
Norma J. Selders, RN
Eleanor Sheridan, RN, BSN, MSN

**20** Oral administration
**36** Tube administration
**50** Rectal administration

## Administering by the parenteral route

CONTRIBUTORS TO
THIS SECTION INCLUDE:
Nancy P. Moldawer, RN, BSN, MSN
Marian Newton, RN, BSN, MN

**62** Parenteral administration
**64** Intradermal administration
**70** Subcutaneous administration
**78** Intramuscular administration
**84** Intravenous administration
**95** Intra-arterial administration

## Administering by the respiratory route

CONTRIBUTORS TO
THIS SECTION INCLUDE:
Susan K. Grove, RN, BSN, MS

**100** Instillation
**108** Inhalation

## Administering by the dermatomucosal route

CONTRIBUTORS TO
THIS SECTION INCLUDE:
Norma J. Selders, RN

**120** Dermatomucosal medications
**121** Skin medications
**132** Eye medications
**140** Ear medications
**144** Mouth and throat medications
**148** Vaginal medications

## Appendices and index

**152** Nurse's guide to dosage calculations
**154** I.V. compatibility chart: Solutions and medications
**155** Acknowledgements
**156** Selected references
**158** Index

# Contributors

*At the time of original publication, these contributors held the following positions.*

**Nancy Burns** is an assistant professor of nursing and director of continuing education at the University of Texas at Arlington School of Nursing. She received her BSN from Texas Christian University in Fort Worth and her MS from Texas Woman's University in Denton, where she's currently a doctoral candidate. In addition to being a member of the American Cancer Society's Texas Division Board of Directors, she belongs to the American Nurses' Association (ANA), the National League for Nursing, the Oncology Nursing Society, and Sigma Theta Tau. She's one of the advisers for this PHOTOBOOK.

**Susan K. Grove,** an assistant professor of nursing at the University of Texas at Arlington School of Nursing, received her BSN from the University of Iowa in Iowa City, and her MS from the University of Oklahoma in Oklahoma City. She's currently a doctoral candidate at Texas Woman's University in Denton, and belongs to the ANA and Sigma Theta Tau.

**Lenora Haston,** also an adviser for this PHOTOBOOK, earned her BSN from Temple University, Philadelphia, Pennsylvania. From 1977 to 1979, she was clinical coordinator for surgery at Temple University Hospital. At present, she's an MSN candidate at the University of Pennsylvania in Philadelphia.

**Nancy P. Moldawer** is an oncology clinical specialist at Temple University Hospital, section of hematology/oncology, in Philadelphia, Pennsylvania. She received her BSN from the University of Michigan in Ann Arbor and her MSN from the University of Pennsylvania in Philadelphia.

**Marian Newton** is an assistant professor at Northeastern University College of Nursing, Boston, Massachusetts. She earned her Associate Degree in Nursing from St. Petersburg (Fla.) Junior College, and her BSN and MN degrees from the University of Florida College of Nursing, in Gainesville. She's a member of the Massachusetts Nurses Association and Sigma Theta Tau.

**Norma J. Selders** is pharmacy head nurse, Technician Training and Management, at Ohio State University Hospitals, Columbus. A graduate of the Miami Valley Hospital School of Nursing, Dayton, Ohio, she's currently a BSN candidate at Ohio University in Athens.

**Eleanor Sheridan** is an assistant professor at Arizona State University College of Nursing in Tempe. After graduating from the Mercy School of Nursing of Detroit (Mich.), she earned her BSN and MSN degrees from Wayne State University College of Nursing, also in Detroit.

# Introduction

**H**ave you ever wondered how to give medication to a gastrostomy patient? How to use a Heaf gun to administer immunotherapy? How to administer medication through an inhalation device? Or how to correctly apply nitroglycerin ointment?

If you have, you know how much you need to learn. Giving medications correctly is not as easy as it sounds. You're responsible for seeing that everything goes right, from patient identification through documentation.

How can you meet such a varied challenge? By reading this PHOTOBOOK. Throughout its pages, you'll find clear, easy-to-understand photostories that'll help you understand all you need to know.

For example, we'll show you the ins and outs of giving oral medications—not just how to administer them, but how to vary that basic procedure for solid or liquid medications, for infants or elderly patients, and for stroke or gastrostomy patients. You'll also see how medications are administered rectally for local or systemic effects.

In another section of this book, you'll learn how to give medications using the parenteral route. This section includes the latest techniques for immunotherapy and intra-arterial therapy. It also features tips on how to inject medication using the Z-track method, and how to read sensitivity test results. And you'll learn about special equipment that's been designed to help the visually impaired diabetic patient.

Are you uncertain about how to administer medications using the respiratory tract? Don't be. Section 4 of this PHOTOBOOK explains how to use everything from a nasal aerosol device (Turbinaire®) to a hand-held nebulizer. If you must teach your patient how to administer his own medication, study the special home care aids. Then copy them on an office copier, and fill in the information relevant to your patient.

Have you noticed the little nursing-cap logos throughout the book? Watch for them. They alert you to helpful nursing tips that'll increase your on-the-job expertise.

As you know, giving medications carries with it big responsibilities. And helping you fulfill these responsibilities is our goal. We think this PHOTOBOOK is the best and most complete guide available. Once you read it, we're sure you'll agree.

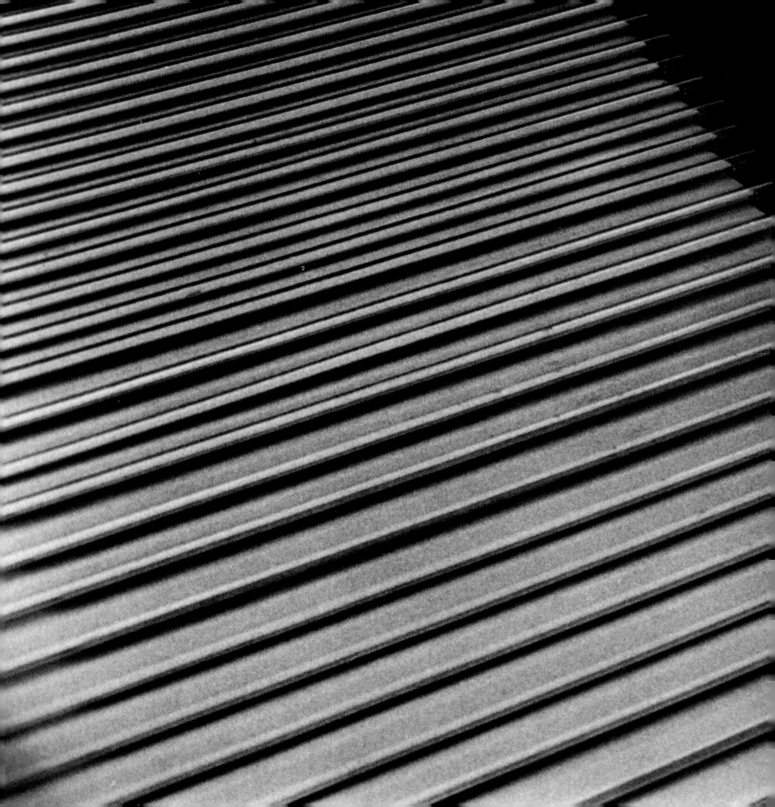

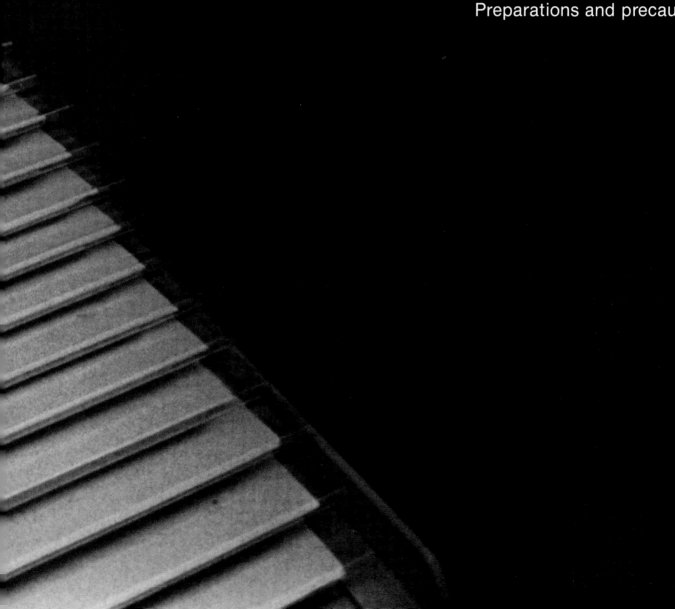

# Beginning the Procedure

Preparations and precautions

# Preparations and precautions

If you're like most nurses, you probably give medication to patients more often than you do any other single task. Perhaps you even consider giving medications the most routine part of your day. But how meticulously do you observe the standard precautions for safe administration? Do you try to save time by not double-checking the drug's name, dosage, and route?

Don't take chances. Read this section carefully to find out how easy it is to make the standard precautions part of your routine. They take less time than you think. And by observing them, you'll not only give medications more efficiently, but also more safely.

## Observing the Five Rights

Before you give *any* medication, compare the doctor's order with the order written on your patient's medication card or Kardex. To do this correctly and efficiently, use the system known as the Five Rights. Ask yourself these questions:
• Right name: Is the patient's *name* the same?
• Right drug: Is the ordered *drug* the same?
• Right dose: Is the ordered *dose* the same?
• Right route: Is the ordered *route* the same?
• Right time and frequency: Is the *time and frequency* of administration the same?

If you find any discrepancy—no matter how small—withhold the medication until you can check with the doctor or pharmacist. Doing so will prevent errors and ensure safe administration.

Here's another important point to remember: Never accept a verbal medication order from anyone, except in an extreme emergency. If such an emergency occurs, write the order on the patient's chart so you can refer to it easily. Then, have the doctor countersign it as soon as possible.

## Taking the necessary precautions

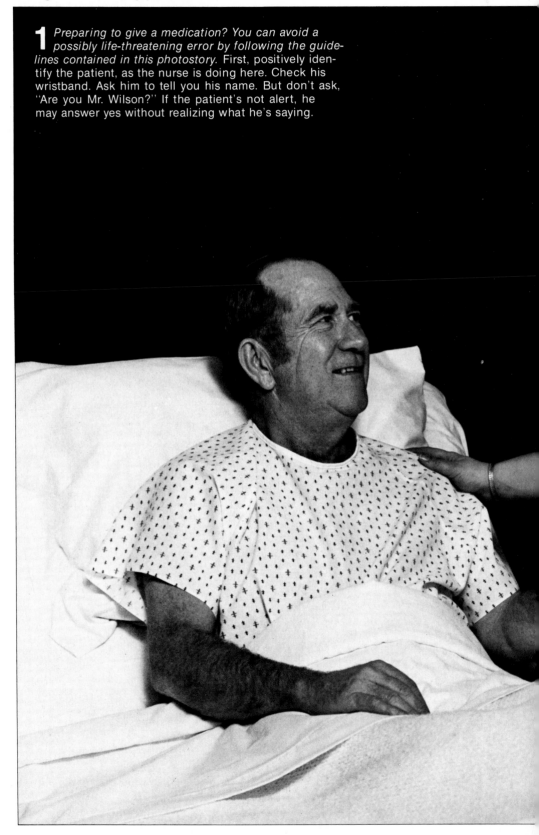

**1** *Preparing to give a medication? You can avoid a possibly life-threatening error by following the guidelines contained in this photostory.* First, positively identify the patient, as the nurse is doing here. Check his wristband. Ask him to tell you his name. But don't ask, "Are you Mr. Wilson?" If the patient's not alert, he may answer yes without realizing what he's saying.

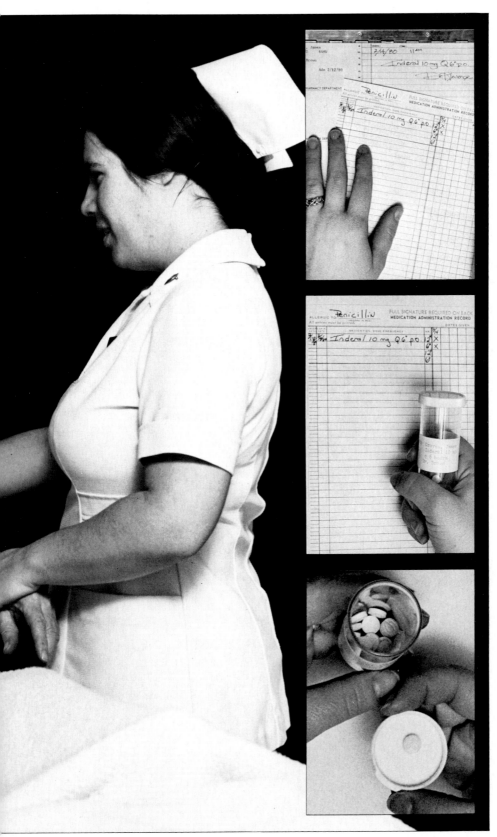

**2** Now, check the doctor's medication order on the patient's chart. Compare the doctor's order with the order written on the patient's medication card or Kardex, using the Five Rights system explained on the opposite page.

Do the orders match? Double-check spelling and abbreviations to make sure you've read them correctly. For example, don't confuse the abbreviation I.M. with I.V., or the drug name digoxin with digitoxin. Check the placement of the decimal points in dosages. If you find any discrepancy, withhold the drug until you can consult the doctor. Then, correct the record and notify the head nurse, so you can complete the appropriate incident report.

**3** If the orders match, use the Five Rights system to check the dispensed *medication* against the Kardex.

Call the pharmacist if you find a discrepancy. However, don't always expect the prescribed dose to match the amount on the medication label. If it doesn't, calculate how many units of the medication you must give to administer the proper dose.

Another important reminder: Check the Kardex for any allergies your patient may have. If the prescribed medication contains a component that the patient's allergic to, withhold the drug until you've consulted the doctor.

**4** Does the dispensed medication match the information on the Kardex? Examine the drug itself. Check the expiration or reconstitution date. Make sure the drug isn't discolored, doesn't smell unusual, and doesn't contain any precipitate (if it's a liquid). If you notice anything amiss, call the pharmacist, and return the medication to him, with an explanation. Then, place a new order.

Let's suppose, however, that everything checks out correctly. Next, consider the questions in the box on page 10. Then, check the medication label once more as you're measuring the dosage. If all's well, you're ready to prepare the patient for administration. Read how in the rest of this section.

# Preparations and precautions

## Using the medication cart

This is a medication cart, which provides the most desirable method for distributing medications. When you use it, expect these benefits:
• You can complete the entire medication procedure, from checking the order to documenting, at each patient's bedside. This makes medication errors less likely.
• The medications to be distributed to other patients are covered and protected from contamination.
• The cart itself can be left in the patient's doorway, reducing the risk of bacteria transfer from one room to another.

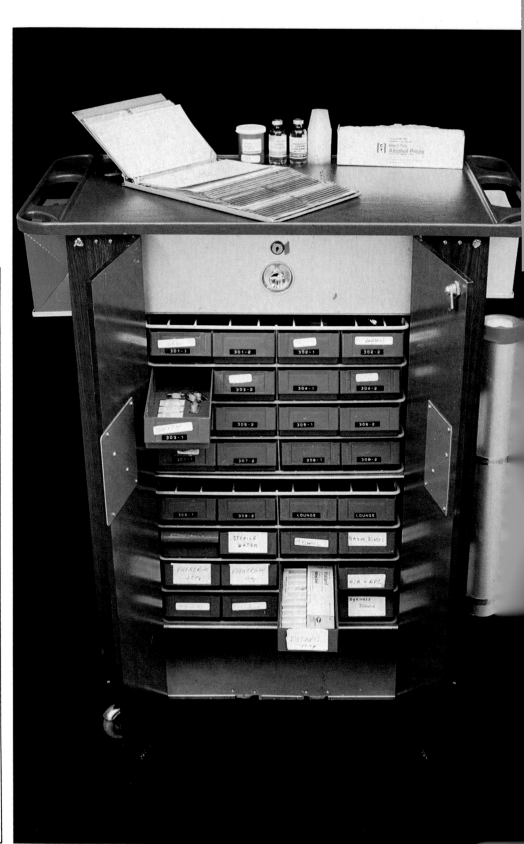

**Know the medication**

Do you know everything you should about the medication you're about to administer? Don't take chances. Ask yourself these questions to properly assess the effects it may have on your patient's condition.
• Is the prescribed medication appropriate for the patient's present or preexisting condition? If it's not, consult the doctor.
• Is the dose within safe limits? If you're not sure, call the pharmacy or consult a drug text; for example, *Nurse's Guide to Drugs*. Then, talk to the doctor.
• Is the ordered route compatible with the patient's condition? For example, if the ordered route is oral and the patient has been vomiting, notify the doctor about the problem. Maybe he'll order the medication in another form.
• Is the medication compatible with other medications the patient is taking? If not, tell the doctor.
• What foods or other medications will affect its absorption? Know this so you can gauge the patient's response to the medication and help determine the cause of any adverse reactions.
• What's the expected effect of the medication? If you're not sure, look it up.
• What are its side effects? Knowing this will make you alert to possible complications.
  Obviously, you can never be too well informed about a drug you're administering. Make information-gathering part of your regular routine.

## Pre-pouring medications

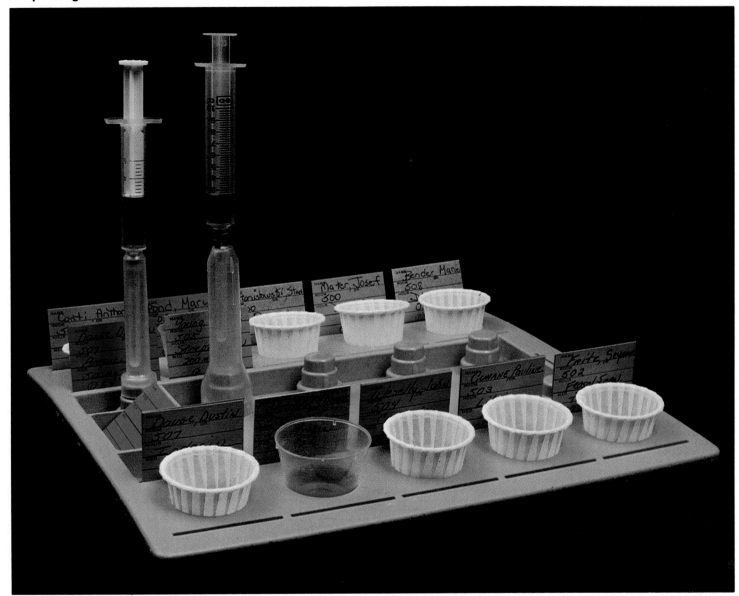

Do you work in a hospital where medication carts aren't used? If you do, you probably pre-pour the medications you give and dispense them from a special tray, such as the one shown here. Take more care than usual if you administer medications this way. Why? Because the pre-pouring method increases the risk of error, as well as the risk of contamination, since you carry the fully loaded tray into each room.

To minimize these hazards, follow these pre-pouring tips carefully:

• Begin by comparing the Kardex with the medication cards and making sure each card is correct. Consult the doctor if you find a discrepancy.

• Wash your hands, and open the medication cabinet. Pour, measure, or draw up the proper dose of medication ordered for each patient. Use souffle cups or disposable medicine cups for all oral medications and suppositories. For medications that must be injected, cap the needles on the syringes.

• Place each dose in its proper spot on the medication tray. Make sure it's directly in front of the slot holding the patient's medication card. Then, pick up the tray and start your rounds.

• When you enter a patient's room, place the medication tray on a flat, stable surface, as far from the patient as possible. This will reduce the risk of contamination.

• After you give each patient his medication, discard his medicine cup immediately (another way to reduce the risk of contamination). Don't touch the rim of the cup or put the empty cup back on the tray. If you've used a syringe, recap it and return it to the tray so you can discard it properly later.

• When you've completed your medication rounds, return to your nursing station. Using the medication cards as guides, immediately chart and document each procedure, following the guidelines on pages 16 and 17. If, for any reason, you didn't give medication to one of your patients, be sure to document why in your nurses' notes.

# Preparations and precautions

## When medication errors aren't reported

You say you know the Five Rights system and all the other rules for giving medications properly. You *know* them, but do you follow them? A recent pharmaceutical study revealed that almost two thirds of all medication errors occur because nurses disregard the Five Rights system.

Yet, errors do occur even when care is exercised. And they're made worse because they go unreported by 3 out of 10 nurses. Why? Perhaps the nurses hate to admit making a mistake. Or maybe they're afraid of losing their jobs. Perhaps they even fear law suits. But these possibilities aren't nearly as bad as what can happen when a medication error isn't reported. This can start a chain reaction of errors, seriously affecting the quality of your patient care. Honesty in reporting medication errors is not only the best policy; it's the most practical one. Consider the following cases:

### The situation
Alma Cheswick, a 69-year-old housewife, has been hospitalized with a pulmonary embolism. As part of her treatment the doctor has ordered 5,000 units of heparin given I.V. every 6 hours. One morning, the nurse who's responsible for distributing medication forgets to administer the heparin to Mrs. Cheswick.

### The nurse's action
To avoid trouble and embarrassment, the nurse charts that she gave Mrs. Cheswick the heparin on schedule.

### The outcome
When routine tests are taken, Mrs. Cheswick's clotting time is recorded at 12 seconds. Naturally, the doctor determines that the clotting time is too fast. He tries to find a reason for it. When he examines the patient's chart and sees that all doses were given as ordered, he increases the heparin dose.

By not reporting her error, the nurse has temporarily escaped reprimand. But in the process, she's increased Mrs. Cheswick's chances of bleeding to death.

*Important:* If you ever forget to give a medication, report the error immediately. Doing otherwise violates your record-keeping responsibilities, the doctor's ability to treat his patient properly, and the patient's right to competent medical care.

### The situation
Charles Schultz, a 53-year-old obese insurance executive, has an intestinal shigella infection. His doctor has ordered 100 mg of doxycycline (Vibramycin*) to be given I.V. every 12 hours, to treat the infection. The nurse on duty misreads the doctor's handwriting, recopies the order on the Kardex incorrectly, and then administers diphenhydramine hydrochloride (Valdrene) instead. That weekend, she looks up Valdrene in a drug text and discovers, to her horror, that it's an antihistamine.

### The nurse's action
Because she's afraid that she will be reprimanded, the nurse decides not to tell Mr. Schultz's doctor about the medication error she made.

### The outcome
When the doctor reviews Mr. Schultz's progress, he assumes that doxycycline is not only ineffective but is causing the patient's urticaria, vomiting and diarrhea, which are side effects of both drugs. He reluctantly begins therapy with ampicillin,* another medication for intestinal shigella, even though it's one that Mr. Schultz had an allergic skin reaction to in postop therapy.

The nurse who made the error has protected herself temporarily but has sacrificed Mr. Schultz's comfort and right to proper medical care.

*Important:* If you ever administer the wrong medication, report your mistake immediately. Your patient's health may depend on it.

*Available in the United States and in Canada.

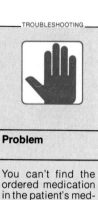

| Problem | |
| --- | --- |
| You can't find the ordered medication in the patient's medication drawer. | |
| You find a medication in the patient's medication drawer, but no order is written on the Kardex. | |
| You notice that the medication does not look the same as it usually does; for example, it's cloudy or a different color. | |
| You discover that the medication container isn't labeled. | |
| Your patient tells you he never received medication like this before. | |

## Administering medications: How to cope with unexpected problems

If you've ever given medications, you know unexpected problems can disrupt normal routine. Study this chart for tips on how to deal with them.

| Possible explanations | Nursing action |
|---|---|
| • An error was detected on the Kardex, so the order was withheld until the doctor could be notified.<br>• The medication was replaced with a generic substitute.<br>• The pharmacy hasn't dispensed the medication yet.<br>• The medication was placed in someone else's bin. | • Go to the order sheet and double-check your information. If this is correct, ask the pharmacy about the medication order. If the order is yet unfilled, or *was* filled (and the medication misplaced), chart the reason why you didn't give the medication. If the medication was replaced with a generic substitute, give that substitute to the patient. |
| • The ordered medication was never transcribed on the Kardex.<br>• The medication was meant for a patient with the same name on another unit.<br>• The medication was discontinued but not removed from the drawer. | • Do not administer the medication until you can go to the order sheet and double-check your information. Then, if it checks out, transcribe the order on the Kardex, and administer the drug. If there's no order for the drug, return it to the pharmacy, with an explanation. |
| • The medication has deteriorated.<br>• The hospital is buying medication in a new generic form.<br>• The wrong medication was placed in the container. | • In such a case, withhold the medication until you can check with the pharmacist. Then, if you don't administer it, chart the reason why. |
| • The label has fallen off. | • Withhold the medication. Then, return the container for relabeling. Document why the medication wasn't administered. |
| • The medication is wrong and was ordered by mistake.<br>• The medication is a new order.<br>• The patient is confused. | • Withhold the medication. Then, if the medication hasn't been ordered, consult with the doctor, and document why you withheld it. If it *has* been ordered, tell your patient the name of the medication and why it was prescribed. |

### Preparing the patient

Let's imagine you're in Mr. Stellankowski's room to give him his morning medications. As he sits in a slumped position, listening to his radio, you follow all the preliminary procedures, including the Five Rights system, on page 8. Once you find everything in order, what do you do next? Ask yourself these questions:

• Is Mr. Stellankowski in the proper position to take his medication? No, he's not. Position him correctly and comfortably.

• Is he familiar with the medication you're giving him? If the medication's new, take time to explain what it is and why the doctor ordered it.

• Do Food and Drug Administration (FDA) regulations require that he read the package insert that came with the medication? If so, provide him with it and make sure he reads it before you give him the first dose. Take time to answer any questions he may have.

• Does the medication involve special administration procedures? If it does, review the procedure. If the patient will give the medication to himself after discharge, share this information with him and a family member. Then, ask him to repeat the instructions to you so you're sure he understands them.

• Does the patient have any other questions about the medication? For example, how long will it take to have an effect? Answer all questions honestly.

Finally, if the patient's taking the medication orally, remain with him until he swallows it.

## Does your patient have an allergy?

You know how important it is to have accurate allergy information when you're administering a drug. But do you always give that information the attention it deserves? You can endanger a patient's life if you administer a drug to which he's allergic. Avoid a serious error like this by following these precautions:

• Anytime you receive a new drug order for your patient, familiarize yourself with the drug's components before administering it.

Take, for example, the nurse who administers Percodan* to the patient with an aspirin allergy. Percodan, as you probably know, contains aspirin. Looking up the drug *before* she administered it could have prevented the patient from developing anaphylactic shock.

• Before giving a patient any drug, check his Kardex in the appropriate space for allergy information.

• If no allergy information is listed on the Kardex, don't assume that the patient has no allergies. Question the patient and his family. Then, if he *does* have an allergy, add the information to his Kardex. If the patient has never received a drug such as penicillin, but several members of his family are allergic to it, assume that he's allergic to penicillin also. Get an order for a substitute antibiotic. If he has no allergies, write: "None known." *Never leave a blank space on this part of the Kardex.*

*Available in the United States and in Canada.

# Preparations and precautions

## You and the law: What are your responsibilities?

"Me? Break the law? Never!" If you're like most nurses, that's probably what you think. But as a nurse you face legal questions every day—and may even break the law without knowing it. Many common hospital situations actually involve ticklish legal questions. Read this page to find out how to deal with them.

**Question:** As a night shift nursing supervisor, you've been called on to dispense drugs from the pharmacy after the pharmacist is no longer on duty. Do nursing laws and pharmacy laws allow you to do this?

**Answer:** Laws differ from state to state, and the legality of this matter is unclear. But most Nursing Practice Acts don't include dispensing medication as a nursing responsibility. Your hospital pharmacy should assume 24-hour responsibility for pharmaceutical functions. If this is impractical, representatives from the pharmacy, the nursing staff, and the administration should draw up a policy covering all concerned parties.

**Question:** You're giving morning medications, and Mr. Chan, in Room 203, refuses to take what's been prescribed for him. What do you do?

**Answer:** Try to find out *why* the patient has refused his medication. Perhaps it makes him ill. For example, maybe he's experiencing some unpleasant side effects that he hasn't told you about. But even with no reason, he has a right to refuse medication. If he does, make sure you chart that the medication wasn't given and why. Then, notify the doctor.

**Question:** Your patient has been getting Demerol* 100 mg I.M. every 4 hours, as necessary, postop a cholecystectomy. He's doing well. When you check him at 3:00 a.m., he says he still has some pain but not as much. You determine he no longer needs 100 mg of Demerol. Instead, you give him 50 mg. Is this the right thing to do?

**Answer:** No. In this case, you should call the doctor and ask him to reduce the dose. By assuming the responsibility yourself and decreasing the dosage, you're practicing medicine without a license, which, as you know, is illegal.

**Question:** A doctor you work with has illegible handwriting. When you politely ask him if he could try writing his medication orders more neatly, he tells you it's your responsibility to be able to read his handwriting, not his. So, the next time you get one of his orders, you don't question it. You simply do your best to decipher the information. If you administer the wrong drug as a result, who's liable?

**Answer:** You're negligent if you carry out an order that you're not sure of; you can be held responsible if the patient suffers an adverse reaction. In the case described above, you should withhold the medication until you can discuss the situation with your supervisor.

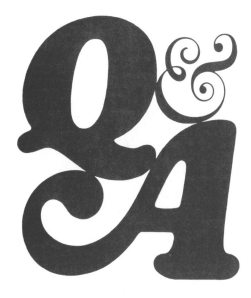

**Question:** A doctor orders both Edecrin* and Coumadin* for your patient, which you know are incompatible and could cause severe bleeding. Do you carry out this order? Who is legally responsible if your patient suffers such a reaction?

**Answer:** You may be, if you carry out an incorrect order. You're considered by law to be a primary health-care provider. Therefore, you're expected to know all about each medication you give; for example, its dosage, indications and contraindications, and its interactions with food and other drugs.

In this case, discuss the order with the doctor, and explain the reason for your concern. If he refuses to change the order, you are within your rights not to give the incompatible drugs.

**Question:** You're a nurse in an oncology unit and one of your patients, a 21-year-old college student, has just died. His family is distraught. The doctor writes an order on the patient's chart to give the patient's mother a tranquilizer. Do you administer the drug? Are you legally protected if you do?

**Answer:** Most hospitals have neglected to write policy on this matter. Without a policy, the safest way to handle the matter is to refer the family member to the emergency department. But if you try to get such a policy written, make sure it not only allows the patient's doctor to write such an order (and authorizes you to follow it), but that it holds the hospital—not you—responsible if the family member has an adverse reaction.

**Question:** You're ordered by a doctor to administer digoxin 0.5 mg I.M. stat. You know that I.M. absorption of digoxin is, at best, unpredictable and, at worst, poor. It's also painful. Do you question the order or do you administer the drug?

**Answer:** You are within your professional and legal bounds to question the order. As a patient advocate, you should not only be concerned about the route's ineffectiveness, but also the unnecessary pain it will cause your patient. Discuss it with the doctor. However, be diplomatic. Then, if he still orders the drug I.M., ask that he administer it himself.

**Question:** You've volunteered to man the first aid station for your church's annual retreat weekend. During this weekend, you administer over-the-counter drugs, patch cuts and bruises, and manage sprains. Does your legal coverage change because of your volunteer status?

**Answer:** It may. So, before you agree to perform such a service, familiarize yourself with the appropriate clauses in your state's Nursing Practice Act and the Good Samaritan law. You may find they differ. Your malpractice insurance *should* cover you whether you're at work or not. A good rule to keep in mind is this: Always practice good nursing principles no matter where you are. Never administer a drug to anyone without knowing his relevant medical history; for example, if he has any drug allergies. Document any special treatment given.

*Available in the United States and in Canada.

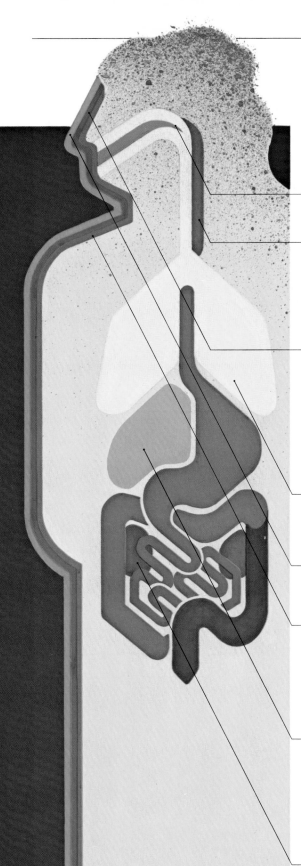

## How a drug's metabolized

When a drug enters the human body, it passes through four basic stages: absorption, distribution, biotransformation, and excretion. This chart explains, in a simplified form, how each stage works.

### Absorption

Mucosa The mucous membrane is the thinnest, most vascular dermal surface, so drug absorption via the mucosa is fairly rapid and effective. The mucous membrane absorbs drugs by diffusion, infiltration, and osmosis. The extent of that absorption varies from one membrane to another.

Gastrointestinal tract Absorption is the transfer of a drug from its entry site to the circulation. Although the safest and easiest route for administering drugs is through the GI tract, drug absorption is unpredictable. Some of the drug dissolves in the stomach. The extent of that dissolution is determined by the size of the drug particles, the pH level of the stomach fluids, and the stomach's contents. But most of the drug is absorbed in the small intestine. The small intestine is best suited for absorption because of its large surface area, its good blood supply, and its pH level of 6 to 8. The pH level makes most drugs nonionic. When this happens, the lipid solubility of the drug increases and absorption occurs.

Parenteral (intradermal, subcutaneous, intramuscular, intravenous, and intra-arterial) Parenteral absorption is not only more reliable than gastrointestinal absorption, but also more rapid. Of the five routes listed above, intradermal absorption is the slowest and is used only for very small doses.

Drugs given subcutaneously are absorbed faster than those given intradermally but slower than those given intramuscularly. Absorption by this route is complete.

Drugs given intramuscularly are also absorbed quickly because of the large surface area and good blood supply of the muscle fibers and fasciae. However, absorption by this route may be incomplete.

Drugs given by intravenous or intra-arterial routes are immediately distributed throughout the patient's system, because they go directly into the bloodstream and bypass the absorption process completely.

Respiratory tract When a drug is given via the respiratory tract, it's absorbed more rapidly and efficiently than it would be in the GI tract, but not as fast as parenterally. Small-particled drugs that are inhaled are transported to the alveoli. There they are absorbed quickly, because of the alveoli's large surface area and good blood supply. Exactly how quickly is determined by the rate and depth of respiration and the drug's ability to permeate the alveolar membrane.

Skin The majority of the drugs applied to the skin are administered for local effects and are not absorbed. The absorption rate of a systemic drug applied to the skin is determined by the density of the drug's base and the thickness of the skin where the drug is applied.

### Distribution

Distribution occurs when a drug binds to plasma protein in the blood and is transported via the circulation to all parts of the body. The drug then crosses cell membranes and enters the body tissue. Some of the drug is also distributed to, and stored in, fat and muscle. Distribution is affected by membrane permeability and blood supply to the absorption area. As the plasma levels in the blood decrease, the drug is released from the tissues, thus maintaining equal drug/blood concentration levels.

### Biotransformation

Biotransformation is the conversion of a drug into a less active and more easily excreted form. Most of this conversion takes place in the patient's liver via synthetic and nonsynthetic reactions. In the synthetic reactions, the hepatic enzymes conjugate the drug with other substances to make it less active. In the nonsynthetic reactions, the drug is oxidized, hydrolyzed, and diffused. These reactions serve to activate, deactivate, or otherwise alter the drug's activity.

Biotransformation takes place in lesser degrees in the kidneys, plasma, and intestinal mucosa. It's slowed in patients with hepatic disease, severe cardiovascular disease, or renal disease.

### Excretion

The drug has effect until it is either changed into an inactive form or is excreted. Excretion of gaseous drugs takes place via the lungs. But most drug excretion is via the kidneys. The kidneys excrete both the pure drug and metabolites of the original drug. They do this via passive glomerular filtration, active tubular secretion, and reabsorption. Factors affecting excretion are the extent of kidney circulation, how much of the drug reaches the kidneys, and rate of glomerular filtration. Drugs are also excreted via the feces, saliva, tears, and in mother's milk.

# Preparations and precautions

**Medications and the elderly**

Is your patient over age 60? If he is, he has a greater chance of reacting adversely to medication than a patient in any other age-group. Indeed, 3% to 5% of all hospital admissions of people over age 60 are because of adverse drug reactions. Every aspect of drug taking—absorption, distribution, biotransformation, action, and elimination—is altered in a body debilitated by age. This slowdown in body functions can unduly prolong drug action or produce toxic levels of the drug in the patient's system. Because of this, an elderly patient may require a greatly reduced dosage of a medication like digitalis,* to avoid toxicity.

To spot a toxic reaction in an elderly patient, make sure you familiarize yourself with the drug he's taking. Learn its side effects, especially those that indicate toxicity.

Don't confuse the signs of toxicity with those of senility. If an elderly patient becomes confused, has trouble concentrating, loses his appetite, or behaves differently, suspect a drug toxicity and notify the doctor.

*Available in the United States and in Canada.

## How to document medications correctly

Record-keeping systems vary from hospital to hospital, so learn the proper way to document medications where you work. Whether you use medication cards, medication Kardexes, or a combination of both, you'll need the following information to complete your records: the patient's name and room number; the date; the medication; dosage; route, frequency, and time of administration; your name and title.

Now, here are some other important guidelines to remember:
• When you're administering a medication by the parenteral route, always record what site you selected for the injection. Doing so will make proper site rotation easier and will prove helpful if problems arise with the injection site. As you can see in the chart to the right, some hospitals assign letters or numbers for easy site identification. Others use abbreviations for body parts; for example, GM for gluteus maximus. They may also use different colored pens to distinguish a change in shifts.
• Never write abbreviations or numbers in a way that might confuse the other health-care professionals who read your notes. For example, never abbreviate the word UNIT. Someone may misread the letter *U* for a poorly written zero and administer an incorrect dose. For doses that contain only fractions of grams, put a 0 *before* the decimal point; for example, 0.25 mg digoxin. Then, no one will misread it for 25 mg.
• Whenever you give a medication, document it as soon as possible. If a drug is ordered but not given, note this on the Kardex, and chart the reason why in your nurses' notes. When you give a medication that's to be administered when needed—such as an analgesic—chart why it was given, whether or not it proved effective, and if it caused any adverse reaction.
• If the patient's drug regimen is discontinued because he's scheduled for surgery, be sure you change the Kardex to indicate this.

### MEDICATION KARDEX

ALLERGIC TO: _Penicillin_
(Record in red)

Dates Given

| Date | Medication, Dose Frequency | Hr. | 1/31 |
|------|----------------------------|-----|------|
| 1/31 | Inderal 10 mg PO Q6° | 12ᴹ | BW |
| | | 6ᴬ | BW |
| | | 12ᴺ | HN |
| | | 6ᴾ | KC |
| 1/31 | Demerol 50 mg IM Q4° PRN chest pain unrelieved by Ntg x2 | 11-7 | 2ᴬᴹ BW / 6ᴬᴹ BW |
| | | 7-3 | |
| | | 3-11 | |
| 1/31 | Ntg gr 1/150 SL PRN chest pain | 11-7 | 1:30ᴬᴹ BW / 1:45ᴬᴹ BW |
| | | 7-3 | |
| | | 3-11 | |

**CODE FOR SITES:**

LA—LEFT ABDOMEN
RA—RIGHT ABDOMEN
LT—LEFT THIGH
RT—RIGHT THIGH
LD—LEFT DELTOID
RD—RIGHT DELTOID
LB—LEFT BUTTOCK
RB—RIGHT BUTTOCK

AGE _68_ RELIGION _J_ DATE ADMITTED _1/31_
DOCTOR _Rose_ INTERN _____
ROOM _203_ NAME _Haag Bernard_
DIAGNOSIS _unstable angina_

DOCUMENTING

Date Discharged _____

S: Subjective Data (symptoms)
O: Objective Data (measurable signs)
A: Assessment (conclusion)
P: Plan Immediate or Future
I: Intervention (procedure or treatment performed)
E: Evaluation (response to intervention)

| Date | Time | No. | Problem | Nursing progress note with signature |
|------|------|-----|---------|--------------------------------------|
| 1/31 | 1³⁰ am | 1 | chest pain | S: Pt. complained of severe substernal chest pain |
|  |  |  |  | O: Diaphoretic. B/P 160/100 HR-132 resp.-28 |
|  |  |  |  | A: angina |
|  |  |  |  | P: relieve pain, monitor VS |
|  |  |  |  | I: O2 applied @ 2L/min. Ntg. gr. 1/150 SL given 1³⁰ am |
|  | 1⁴⁵ am |  |  | S: 1⁴⁵ am pain unrelieved |
|  |  |  |  | I: Ntg gr. 1/150 SL repeated |
|  |  |  |  | O: B/P - 160/110 HR-140 |
|  |  |  |  | S: pain continues |
|  |  |  |  | I: B/P-150/110, HR-120, resp-24 |
|  | 2 am |  |  | I: EKG done. Demerol 50 mg. IM given LB |
|  | 2²⁰ am |  |  | O: B/P-130/90, HR-88 resp.-20 |
|  |  |  |  | E: pain relieved VS returned to normal, no diaphoresis resting comfortably |
|  |  |  |  | Bonnie Weaver, RN. |

ANOTHER PAGE IS IN USE CHECK HERE IN RED ☐

AM 12 | 1 | 2 | 3 | 4 | 5 | ⑥ | 7 | 8 | 9 | 10 | 11

PM 12 | 1 | 2 | 3 | 4 | 5 | ⑥ | 7 | 8 | 9 | 10 | 11

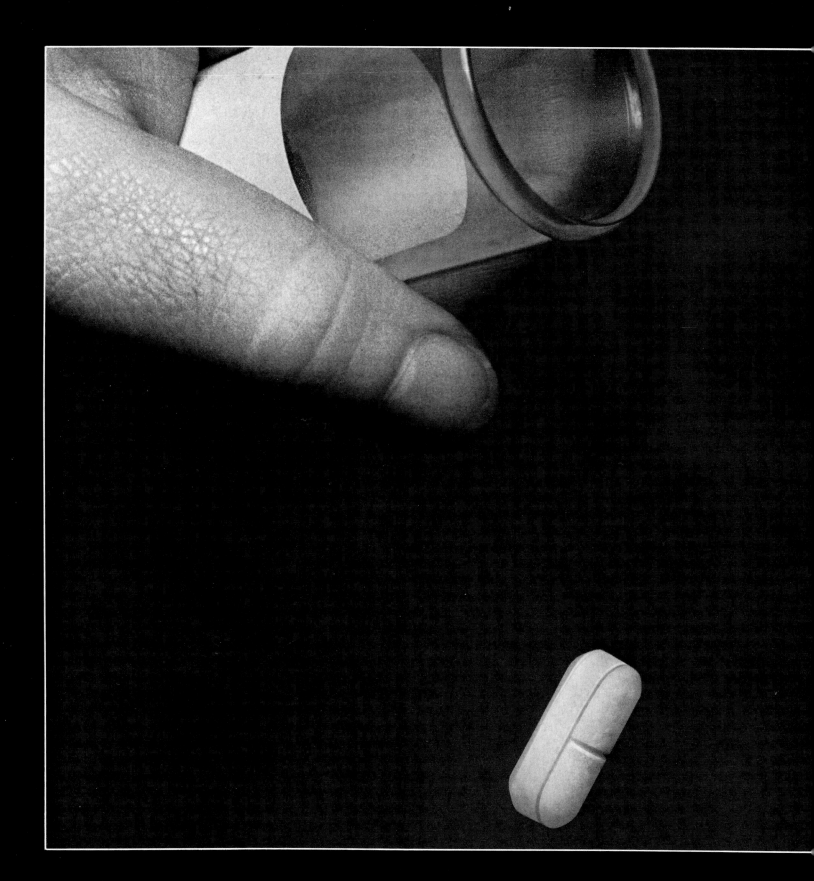

# Administering by the Gastrointestinal Route

Oral administration
Tube administration
Rectal administration

# Oral administration

Doctors prescribe oral medications more than any other kind. So, you may give them every day. But do you really know all you should about them? For example, do you understand how drugs are absorbed in the GI tract? Do you know when you may open a capsule and mix its contents with food or beverages—and when it's downright dangerous to do so? Can you give oral medication to an infant or a stroke victim safely? And what about the patient who's about to go home—how can you help him comply with his medication schedule?

On the following pages, you'll learn the answers to these questions, and more. You'll discover many nursing tips for helping patients with special problems. You may even learn answers to questions you've never considered before.

## How oral medication's absorbed in the GI tract

You probably give oral medications every day. But chances are you don't know much about what happens to them after the patient swallows them. We won't try to cover every aspect of how medication enters your patient's bloodstream. But you can brush up on the basics by examining the illustrations below and reading the questions and answers that follow.

• *What factors influence a solid medication's dissolution rate?* The method of disintegration, for starters. Chewable tablets, for example, dissolve more quickly than those swallowed whole. Another factor is the particle size of the disintegrated medication. In most cases, small particles of medication dissolve in the gastric fluids more quickly than large particles. A third factor

influencing the dissolution rate is the type and amount of filler (inert substances) contained in the tablet or capsule.

• *Is the pH of the medication important?* Definitely. Acidic medications are more soluble in the alkaline fluids of the small intestine; alkaline medications are more soluble in the acidic fluids of the stomach.

• *I know that gastric emptying moves the stomach contents into the small intestine. But what determines the rate of gastric emptying?* A variety of factors, among them the patient's hormonal activity; his physical activity; and the volume, temperature, and pH of his stomach contents. Even his body position's important.

• *How can I position the patient's body to affect gastric emptying?* You can encourage

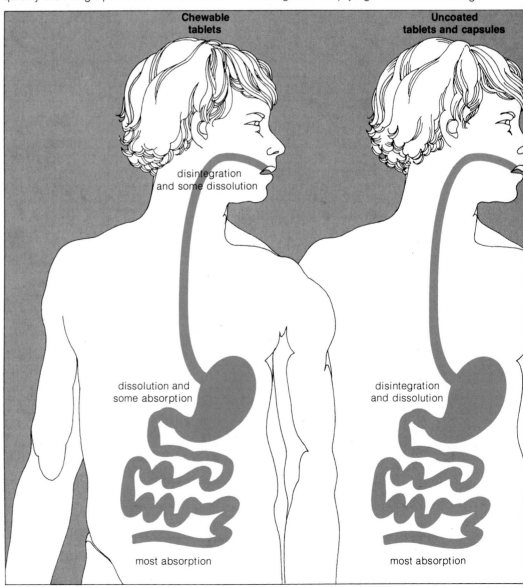

**Chewable tablets**

disintegration and some dissolution

dissolution and some absorption

most absorption

**Uncoated tablets and capsules**

disintegration and dissolution

most absorption

*quick* gastric emptying by seating your patient upright or placing him on his right side. But what if you want to *slow* gastric emptying; for example, when you give a patient an antacid to treat stomach distress? Position him on his *left* side to keep the antacid in his stomach longer.

● *How does the patient's peristaltic rate affect absorption?* An increased peristaltic rate, such as that caused by diarrhea, can decrease absorption by moving the medication through the small intestine too quickly. As a result, a patient suffering from diarrhea may absorb his oral medication poorly.

● *Should I give medication with meals or between meals?* That depends. Food can protect the gastric mucosa from irritation.

However, a full stomach may also slow the absorption rate or alter the medication's therapeutic qualities. The only way to be sure is to check the special considerations and incompatibilities for each medication you give.

● *Can particular foods change a medication's therapeutic qualities?* They certainly can. Some penicillins, for example, decompose prematurely when mixed with fruit juices. Griseofulvin, however, isn't absorbed completely unless the patient takes it with fatty foods.

● *What's the advantage of diluting medication with a beverage like orange juice?* Dilution may actually enhance absorption, provided the medication and the beverage are compatible.

## Ensuring proper absorption

Because the factors affecting drug absorption are so complex, you must take certain measures to make sure a medication's absorbed properly. Consider these questions as you give oral medications:

● *Is your patient taking any other medication?* If he is, make sure all medications are compatible.

● *Should you give the medication with a meal, or when the patient's stomach is empty?* That depends on the medication. But remember, whenever you give medication with a meal, you must find out which foods (if any) to avoid or include.

● *Has the doctor substituted a liquid dose for a solid one?* If so, he may have to alter the dosage as well.

● *Are you substituting one brand of tablet or capsule for another brand of the same medication?* Review the prescription with the pharmacist whenever you change brands of medication. Remember, the change in filler material may so alter the rate of dissolution and absorption that the drug would fail to be therapeutic or possibly even prove toxic.

● *Does the patient have any disease or condition, such as gastroenteritis, that could inhibit oral drug absorption?* If he does, check with the doctor. He may choose another route of administration.

*Important:* After you give any medication, watch your patient to see if the medication has the intended effect. Remember, any patient may react adversely to a medication. If your patient does, notify the doctor immediately.

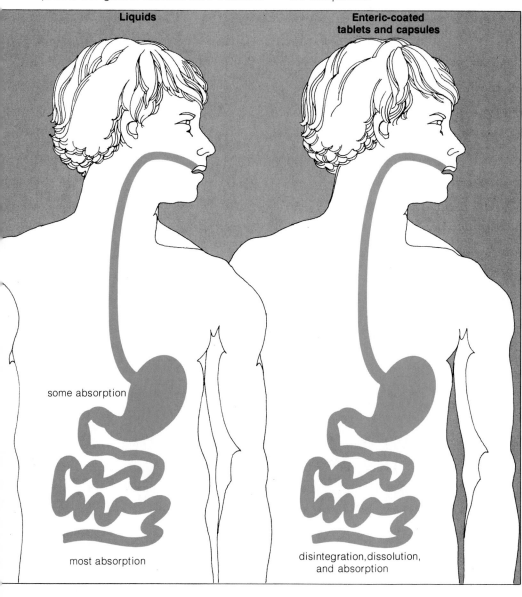

**Liquids**

some absorption

most absorption

**Enteric-coated tablets and capsules**

disintegration, dissolution, and absorption

# Oral administration

## Oral drugs: Some important considerations

### Advantages
- Simple and convenient. In most cases, the patient can take the drug himself.
- Safe. In case of overdose, gastric lavage or vomiting may be used to retrieve or dilute drug.
- Economical.

### Disadvantages
- The relatively slow absorption rate makes the oral route unsuitable for most emergencies.
- Drug effectiveness is somewhat unpredictable. The amount of drug circulating in the patient's system can vary, depending on how well it was absorbed in the GI tract.
- Some oral drugs may irritate the GI tract. Others may discolor the teeth or have an unpleasant taste.
- If the patient is combative or debilitated, he may accidentally aspirate an oral drug.
- Oral drugs may not be suitable for all patients; for example, those with a history of drug abuse or those who may not be capable of managing their own therapy. Oral drugs are also dangerous to have in households where there are small children.

## Getting acquainted with tablets and capsules

You don't have to be a nurse to know something about tablets and capsules. Nearly everyone has taken medication in these forms at one time or another. Because tablets and capsules are stable, in predetermined accurate doses, and easy to use, they're the most frequently prescribed type of medication. Many of them—for example, aspirin—are readily available without prescription.

But, as a nurse, you need to know much more about tablets and capsules than most people do. In the preceding section, you learned the general guidelines for giving *any* medication safely. But what about the specifics? For example, do you know when you can safely open a capsule and mix its contents with food? Or when you can divide a tablet and give it in portions? Read what follows for the background you need to answer correctly.

### Learning about tablets
Tablets come in a wide variety of shapes, colors, and sizes, and may be shaped by either compression or molding. In addition to the medication itself, they may include one or more of these ingredients:

- diluents, such as lactose, starch, or dextrose, to add bulk and ensure proper size and consistency
- disintegrants, such as starch, to speed the disintegration and dissolution process
- coatings, to add color, disguise an unpleasant taste, protect the gastric mucosa from irritation, and protect the tablet from air, light, and moisture. An enteric coating allows the tablet to pass through the stomach intact and dissolve in the small intestine.

Some uncoated tablets are scored for easy division. You may cut or break them into halves or quarters if the dosage calls for only a portion of a tablet. *Important:* Never divide a tablet that's *not* scored. Why? Because you can't be sure the dosage will be accurate unless the tablet's been marked for this purpose by the manufacturer. If an unscored tablet isn't available in the appropriate size, review the prescription with the doctor.

### Learning about capsules
Like tablets, capsules come in a variety of colors, shapes, and sizes. Lengths range from 12 mm (a number 5 capsule) to 28 mm (a number 000 capsule).

The medication in a capsule may be in one of a variety of forms: powders, granules, oils, or liquids other than oil. Usually, the medication is mixed with one or more diluents, solvents, or other pharmacologically inert substances. Solid medication particles may be coated with substances that permit sustained release of small amounts of medication over a prolonged period of time.

After mixing, the medication is encased in a thin shell, usually made of gelatin. This gelatin shell disintegrates quickly in gastric fluids, releasing the medication, which is then absorbed in the GI tract. Since capsule medication is already in liquid or particle form, it's usually absorbed faster than medication compressed into tablet form.

Although most capsules have thin gelatin shells, some have shells made of harder gelatin. And a few have sustained release or enteric coatings, although these are unusual.

### Mixing solid medications with food or beverages
Suppose your patient has difficulty swallowing. You may

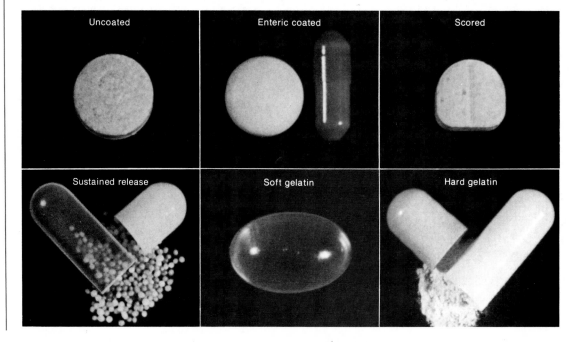

| Uncoated | Enteric coated | Scored |
| Sustained release | Soft gelatin | Hard gelatin |

want to crush a tablet or open a capsule to make administration easier. When is it safe to do this?

As a rule, you may crush uncoated tablets and open soft, uncoated capsules. Then you can mix the medication in a beverage or a small amount of soft food, like applesauce or mashed potatoes, before administering it. *Important:* Before mixing any medication with food or a beverage, make sure the drug's action won't be affected. And since the medication may change the food's taste, always tell the patient what you've done.

Now, here are some tablets and capsules that must *never* be crushed or opened:
• coated tablets and hard or coated capsules. A coating or hard gelatin shell makes swallowing easier and may disguise an unpleasant taste. And remember, an enteric coating keeps the tablet or capsule intact until it reaches the small intestine, where the coating is dissolved in the alkaline secretions and the drug is released. If you destroy the coating, the drug won't be absorbed properly.

*Important:* Tell the patient not to chew coated tablets. Give enteric-coated tablets and capsules with plenty of water when the patient's stomach is empty, to assure quick passage into his small intestine. Never give enteric-coated tablets with milk or antacids, or they'll disintegrate prematurely.
• prolonged-action and repeat-action capsules. Opening and administering these capsules may alter dosage, thus increasing the risk of overdose.

**Storing tablets and capsules**
Protect tablets and capsules from humidity, light, and air. Signs of deterioration include discoloration and unusual odor. Return any medication that looks or smells strange to the pharmacy. Also, check the expiration date and discard medication that's outdated.

## Giving tablets and capsules

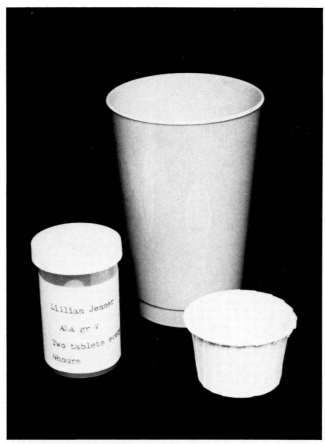

**1** *Before you administer any medication, double-check the medication label with the doctor's order. Then, confirm the patient's identity by checking her wristband and asking the patient her name. Finally, wash your hands thoroughly, and remember to maintain clean technique throughout the procedure. Now, you're ready to begin.*

First, gather the equipment. If you plan to crush an uncoated tablet, you'll need a mortar and pestle or a commercially made pulverizer; if you plan to divide a scored tablet, you'll need a knife. But most of the time, all you'll need is the bottle of medication, a small souffle cup or medicine cup, and water or juice.

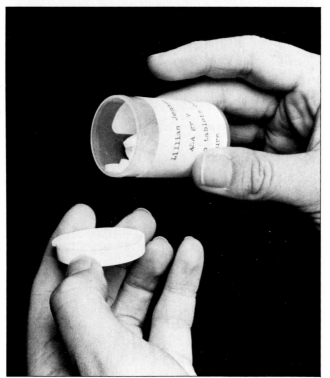

**2** Pour the correct number of tablets or capsules into the bottle cap. If you pour out too many, put the excess back. *Important:* Never touch any of the excess medication or you may contaminate the entire bottle. For the same reason, don't return the unused portion of a divided tablet to the bottle. Instead, discard it.

# Oral administration

**Giving tablets and capsules** continued

**3** Now, pour the tablets or capsules into the souffle cup or medicine cup, and recap the medication bottle. Then, give the cup to the patient or tap the medication into her hand. Keep the water or juice nearby.

*Nursing tip:* If your patient has trouble swallowing tablets or capsules, instruct her to drink some of the water or juice *before* she takes the medication.

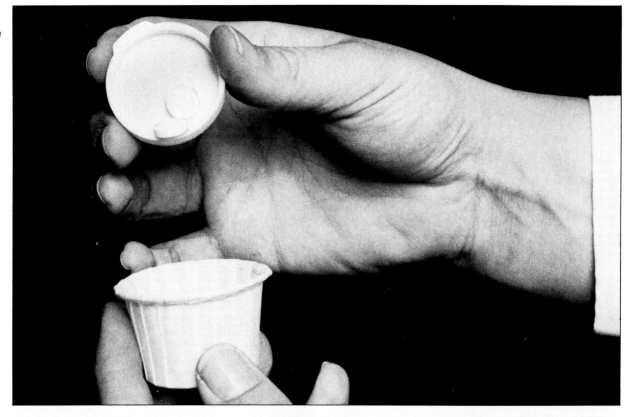

**4** Now, tell the patient to put the tablets or capsules well back on her tongue. (She may take them one at a time or all at once, whichever way she prefers.) If she can't do this herself, help her.

*Important:* Avoid touching the patient's mouth, or the rim of the medicine cup after she's used it. If you do, wash your hands immediately, so you don't transfer any bacteria to your next patient.

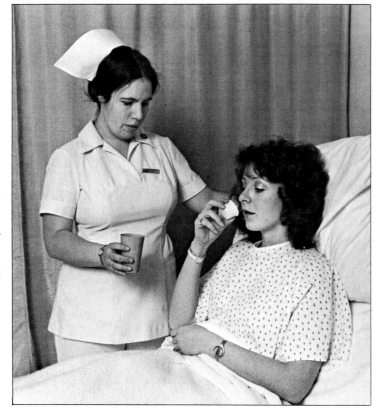

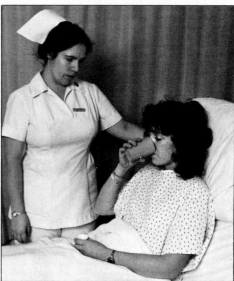

**5** Then, ask her to tip her head slightly forward, and swallow a full mouthful of water or juice. Warn her not to throw her head back as she swallows. This position may prevent her airway from closing and may increase the risk of aspiration.

Finally, discard the used souffle cup and document the procedure according to the guidelines on pages 16 and 17.

## Learning about liquid oral medications

| Type | Description | Nursing considerations |
|------|-------------|------------------------|
| **Syrup** | • A drug and preservative in a viscous, sugar/water solution; usually flavored | • When giving a syrup for a demulcent (soothing) effect, don't follow it with water. Tell the patient to sip the syrup slowly.<br>• When giving a syrup for a systemic effect, you may dilute it. However, dilute only the dose being given. If you dilute the entire bottle, you may destroy the preservative and hasten contamination or decomposition.<br>• Use caution when administering syrups to diabetic patients. Check with the pharmacist to see if a sugar-free syrup is available.<br>• When giving syrups with other drugs, be sure to administer syrups *last*.<br>• Remember, take special care to keep syrups out of the reach of children. |
| **Suspension** | • *Magma:* a thick, milky suspension of an insoluble (or partly soluble) inorganic drug, suspended in water<br>• *Gel:* the same as magma but with smaller drug particles<br>• *Emulsion:* droplets of fat or oil, suspended in water | • Always shake a suspension thoroughly before giving it.<br>• If desired, you may dilute most suspensions with water before administration. However, don't dilute an *antacid* suspension, or it won't coat the stomach effectively. |
| **Alcoholic solution** | • *Elixir:* a mixture of drugs, alcohol, water, and sugar; sweet-tasting. However, elixirs are not as sweet as syrups. They are also less viscous than syrups. Alcohol concentration ranges from 10% to 40% (0.1 to 0.4 g of drug per ml of solution).<br>• *Spirits:* a solution of volatile substances; for example, liquids, solids, or gases. The alcohol in the solution acts as a preservative and solvent. Drug concentration ranges from 5% to 20% (0.05 to 0.2 g of drug per ml).<br>• *Tincture:* a solution of alcohol, or alcohol and water, with drugs. Drug concentration ranges from 10% to 20% (0.1 to 0.2 g of drug per ml).<br>• *Fluidextract:* a bitter solution of vegetable drugs, usually sweetened with a syrup or flavoring. Fluidextracts are rarely prescribed, because they are unusually potent and unpleasant tasting. Drug concentration is 100% (1 g of drug per ml). | • Check the solution carefully. Never administer one that has precipitate at the bottom of the bottle.<br>• If the dose is over 5 ml, double-check it.<br>• If you want to dilute the solution, use only a small amount of water. More water could cause the drug to precipitate.<br>• Consult the pharmacist before you mix alcoholic solutions with liquids other than water. Mixing with other liquids may be contraindicated.<br>• Follow administration with water, unless the solution's given for cough relief.<br>• Store solution in an airtight container. Protect from temperature extremes. Protect fluidextracts from light.<br>• Use these solutions cautiously if your patient is an alcoholic. *Important:* Never give an alcoholic solution to a patient receiving Antabuse. |
| **Reconstituted powders and tablets** | • Solid drugs reconstituted with water (or another suitable liquid) and given to the patient in suspension or solution form | • Read the directions carefully before reconstituting powders and tablets. Don't use too much water with effervescent tablets or they'll boil out of the glass.<br>• Some powders will become gelatinous very quickly after you mix them. Administer them immediately after reconstitution.<br>• Wait until effervescent tablets dissolve completely before you give them to the patient. Give without further dilution. |

# Oral administration

**Measuring liquid medication in a disposable medicine cup**

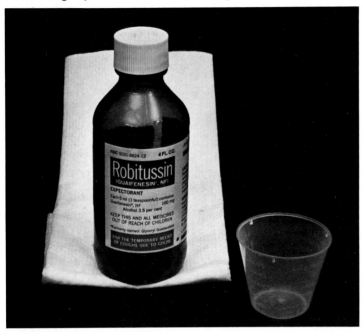

**1** *After you confirm the doctor's order, wash your hands, and properly identify the patient, you're ready to measure the prescribed dosage of liquid oral medication. If you're using a disposable medicine cup, here's how:*

To begin, you'll need the bottle of medication, a disposable medicine cup like the one you see here, and a damp paper towel. If you plan to dilute the medication, also obtain some water or juice. (However, make sure the medication's compatible with the diluent.)

Choose a disposable medicine cup that has all the markings you need. Never try to estimate measurements *between* markings, or your dosage won't be accurate. Check the bottle label against the Kardex.

Is the medication a suspension? Shake it well. Then, uncap the bottle, and place the cap upside down on a clean surface.

Rinse the medication cup in water. This will prevent medication from sticking to its sides.

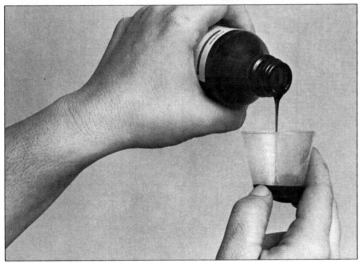

**2** Locate the correct marking on the medicine cup. Keeping your thumbnail on the mark, hold the cup at eye level, and pour in the correct amount of medication.

🐟 *Nursing tip:* As you pour, keep the label pointed up, so spilled liquid won't obscure it. Recheck the label against the Kardex.

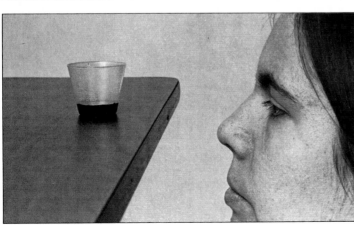

**3** Now, recheck the dosage you've poured into the cup. To do this, set the cup on a level surface, and read the base of the meniscus at eye level. If you've poured too much medication into the cup, discard the excess. Don't return it to the bottle.

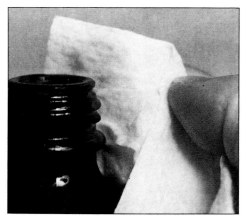

**4** Wipe the bottle lip with a damp paper towel, taking care not to touch the inside of the bottle. Replace the cap. Recheck the label against the Kardex.

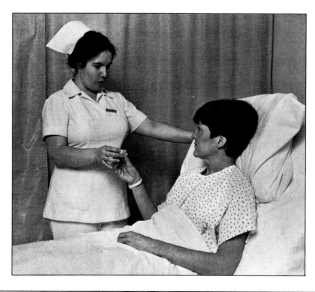

**5** Now you're ready to give the medication to the patient. Position her comfortably in either a sitting or high Fowler's position. Hand her the cup of medication, and wait until she drinks it all. *Important:* Some medications, such as liquid iron preparations and hydrochloric acid, stain the teeth. Administer these by placing a straw toward the back of the patient's mouth. Follow the medication with water.

Discard the medicine cup, taking care not to touch the rim and contaminate your fingers. Finally, document the entire procedure according to the guidelines on pages 16 and 17.

## Giving medication with a medication syringe

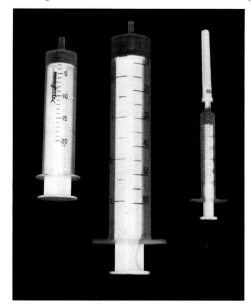

**1** *What if you must give liquid medication to a patient who can't drink from a cup; for example, someone with a fractured jaw? Administer it with a medication syringe. Here's how:*

As you see in this photo, syringes vary in size. Some are marked in teaspoons as well as cubic centimeters or milliliters, and most are disposable. When choosing a syringe, consider the size of the dose, and the size and age of the patient. Always select a syringe that's marked precisely for your needs. Never try to estimate between markings.

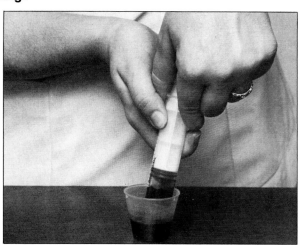

**2** How can you avoid contaminating the medication bottle with the syringe? First, pour the medication into a medicine cup. Then, withdraw the prescribed amount from the cup, with the syringe. Discard the cup and any excess medication. Never return medication to the bottle.

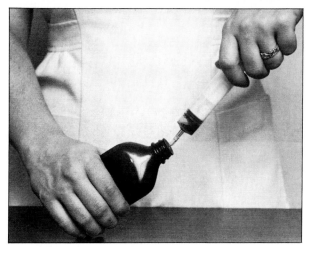

**3** Or try this alternative. Put a sterile needle on the syringe, and withdraw the prescribed amount directly from the bottle. Then, discard the needle. (To learn how to withdraw medication using a Baxa Bottle Adaptor, see page 29.)

# Oral administration

**Giving medication with a medication syringe** continued

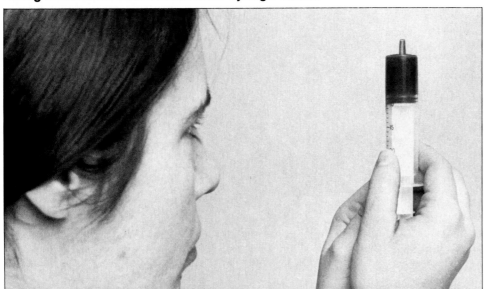

**4** Now, check the dosage. Hold the syringe at eye level, and read the measurement from the top edge of the rubber stopper, as the nurse is doing here. If you've withdrawn too much, squirt the excess into a sink or wastebasket. Don't return it to the bottle.

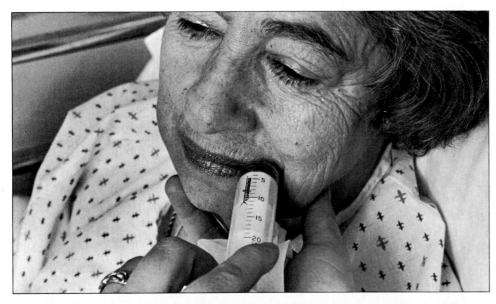

**5** Get ready to give the medication to your patient. Seat her upright or place her in a high Fowler's position. To minimize aspiration risk, place the syringe tip in the pocket between her cheek mucosa and her second molar. Instill the medication slowly. Then, discard the syringe, and document the procedure.

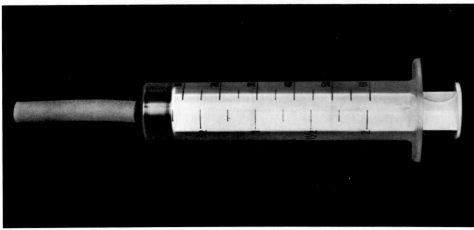

**6** Are you using a large-volume (50 cc or more) syringe? To ease administration, place a 2" (5 cm) length of latex tubing on the syringe tip. Then, you can easily instill medication into the cheek pocket without putting the entire syringe into the patient's mouth. You'll find that this improvised syringe tip is especially handy for elderly, confused, or severely debilitated patients.

Remember, most large-volume syringes are reusable. Wash and rinse them thoroughly after each use.

## How to use the Baxa Bottle Adaptor and Dispensor

**1** *Want to know another way to measure liquid doses of medication without contaminating the bottle? Use the Baxa Bottle Adaptor shown here. This simple device allows you to withdraw medication directly from the bottle, with a special medication syringe, the Baxa Oral Liquid Dispensor. To use it, follow these steps:*

First, open the medication bottle, and make sure the bottle neck is clean and dry.

[Inset] Then, using both thumbs, press the narrow end of the adaptor into the bottle.

Does it fit snugly? If it doesn't, try remedying this by removing the adaptor and rinsing it with warm water; then, try again.

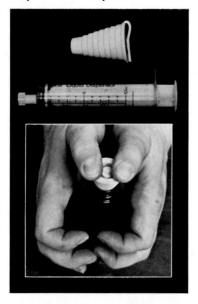
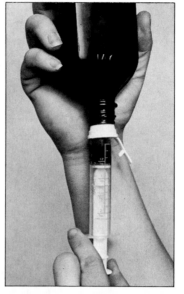

**2** When the adaptor is *securely* in the bottle, open the cap. Then, remove the protective cap from the dispensor, and insert the dispensor into the adaptor, as shown here.

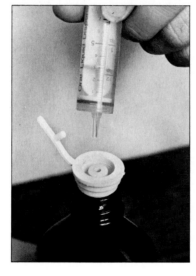

**3** Now, invert the entire unit, and withdraw the prescribed amount of medication. To ensure accuracy, make sure you're at eye level with the top edge of the rubber stopper on the dispensor's plunger.

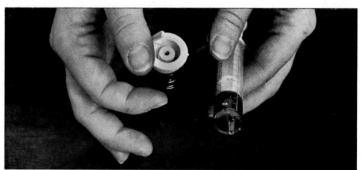

**4** Place the bottle right side up, remove the dispensor, and recap the adaptor. Squirt the medication into a cup, and give it to your patient. Is your patient an infant, or an adult with a fractured jaw? Put the medication directly into his mouth, as shown on page 28.

In any case, when the medication's used up, you may transfer the adaptor to another bottle only if it's for the same patient.

---

SPECIAL CONSIDERATIONS

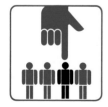

### Giving unpalatable medications

Does the liquid medication you're giving have an unpleasant taste? Make it more palatable for your patient by using one or more of these tips:
• Disguise the taste of the medication by diluting it with water, juice, or Coke™ syrup. But first, make sure the medication's compatible with the other liquid.
• Give the medication with a syringe. Bypass the patient's tastebuds by instilling the medication into the pocket between his cheek and the second molar.
• Ask the patient to suck ice chips to numb his tastebuds before he takes the medication.

• Pour the medication over ice, and give it through a straw. However, avoid this method if you're giving a small dose, because it may affect accuracy.
• If the medication's oily, chill it first. Store oily medications in a refrigerator, unless contraindicated.
• Suggest that the patient hold his nose as he swallows.
• Minimize a bitter aftertaste by offering the patient hard candy or chewing gum after the medication. Or suggest that he gargle, or rinse his mouth with water or mouthwash.

# Oral administration

## Giving medication to an infant

**1** *Any oral medication you administer to an infant will be liquid and prescribed in very small doses. Use a dropper to ensure accuracy. Here's how:*

First, put a bib under the infant's chin and a towel over your shoulder. Then, position the infant in the crook of your arm, as the nurse is doing here. Hold him so his head is elevated at a 45° angle. If necessary, use one of your hands to restrain his arms.

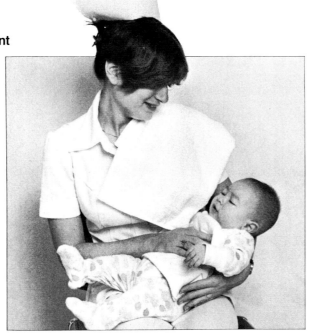
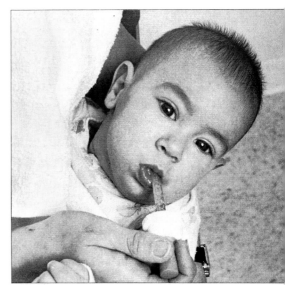

**2** With your other hand, withdraw the correct amount of medication from the bottle by squeezing the bulb on the dropper.

If the dropper's calibrated, check the dose by holding it vertically and looking at it from eye level. Squeeze any excess into a sink or wastebasket. Don't return it to the bottle.

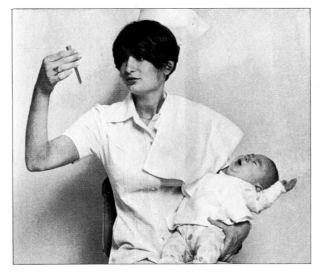
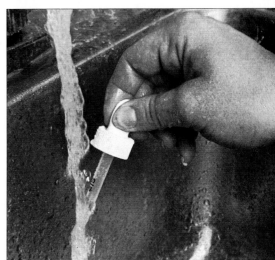

**3** Now, get ready to instill the drops. If the infant won't open his mouth, try pinching his cheek gently.

If the dropper's not calibrated, hold it vertically over the infant's open mouth, and instill the prescribed number of drops.

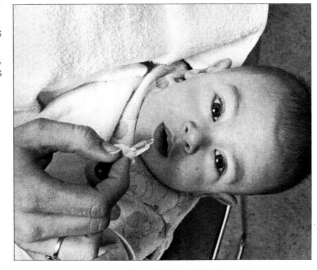
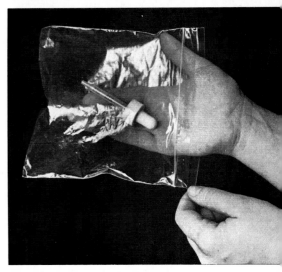

SPECIAL CONSIDERATIONS

**Giving medications: Special considerations**

**4** If you're using a calibrated dropper, instill the medication into the pocket between the infant's cheek and his gum. Putting the medication in that spot will keep him from spitting it out and also reduce the risk of aspiration.

**5** If the dropper touches the inside of the infant's mouth, consider it contaminated. Wash the dropper thoroughly with soap and water; then, rinse and dry it.

**6** Suppose you've prevented contamination. If the dropper's attached to the bottle cap, simply return it to the bottle and screw the cap on tightly. But if it's unattached, rinse the medication out of it with warm water, put it in a clean plastic bag, and store it with the infant's medication bottle. Document the procedure.

*Important:* Never use the same dropper for more than one patient. Keep each infant's dropper separate and labeled with his name. Dispose of the dropper when the medication's gone.

### When your patient's a child

Suppose your patient has just reached school age. Although he probably can swallow a tablet or capsule safely, he may be more willing to take a sweet-tasting syrup or chewable tablet. Avoid problems by finding out if the medication's available in either of these forms.

Avoid giving your patient an elixir, because he'll probably dislike the alcohol flavor. But if you must, remember to dilute it first with a small amount of water.

Encourage his cooperation by acting as if you expect it. However, if he balks, don't threaten or embarrass him. And never insist that he swallow a medication. Doing so may cause him to aspirate the medication.

When giving a young patient medication, keep these pointers in mind:
• Avoid mixing medication with food. If the child detects a strange taste, he may refuse that particular dish in the future.
• When you know medication won't taste good, tell him. Don't try to trick a child. Doing so will make him less cooperative next time. (For tips on how to make medication taste better, read page 29.)
• Never tell a child that medication's candy. He may look for an opportunity to eat or drink the entire contents of the bottle.
• Praise him for his cooperation, if you get it. Let him keep the medicine cup as a trophy, but be sure to rinse it out first.

### When your patient's a stroke victim

If your patient's ability to swallow is seriously impaired, giving oral medication isn't safe. But what if he's a stroke patient and only one side of his head and body is affected? If he's alert and cooperative, with your help he may be able to swallow oral medication.

Before you begin, remember that your patient's stroke has probably affected him in many ways. Keep this in mind when you give him his medication. For example, if the vision on his impaired side is affected, approach and treat him from his unimpaired side, so he can see what you're doing. If he suffers from some form of aphasia, speak to him slowly, explaining the procedure to him in words he can understand. Don't bombard him with information or you may confuse him. Speak calmly and reassuringly.

How can you help a stroke patient swallow medication safely? Try to give him the medication in solid form, because a textured substance is easier for him to control than a liquid. Crush uncoated tablets or open soft capsules, and mix them with a soft food, like applesauce or mashed potatoes. However, never mix the medication with a milk product. Milk products will stimulate salivation, which will increase the risk of aspiration.

*Nursing tip:* If your patient's afraid of choking on his medication, place the fingers of his unim-

paired hand on his neck. When he feels his neck muscles working as he swallows, his confidence may be restored. To be perfectly safe, however, have suctioning equipment handy.

Minimize the risk of aspiration in any stroke patient by following this procedure:
• When you're giving him medication or food, put it on the back of his tongue, on the *unimpaired* side of his mouth. Then, gently turn his head toward the unimpaired side. *Important:* Never tilt his head backward. This position makes aspiration more likely.
• Give him a sip of water, and ask him to swallow. At the same time, press lightly on the *impaired* side of his neck, to stimulate the swallowing reflex. Continue to give him small sips of water until he's swallowed the food or medication. Then, check his mouth. Remove any food or medication trapped on his impaired side.
• Finally, document the entire procedure. Record foods that seem to give your patient particular trouble. For example, if he has difficulty swallowing applesauce, make a note on his care plan and medication Kardex not to mix his medication with applesauce the next time.

As always, use your own judgment. If you think giving oral medication's too risky for your patient, tell the doctor. He may choose another route.

### When your patient has a tracheostomy

Be especially careful when you're giving medication to a patient with a cuffed tracheostomy tube. First, make sure the cuff's inflated, because the inflated cuff blocks off the trachea around the outer cannula, preventing aspiration. However, if the patient has a trach talk-attachment, replace it with a T-piece *before* you inflate the cuff. Otherwise, he won't be able to exhale.

Don't rush when you give the patient his medication. If he coughs or chokes, stop what you're doing immediately. Then wait until he's calm before you continue. Finally, minimize the risk of aspiration by suctioning the trachea before deflating the cuff. Tell the doctor if the patient had difficulty swallowing the medication.

Document the entire procedure.

# Oral administration

## Preparing the patient for home care

If you've ever worked as a visiting nurse, you probably know that once a patient's discharged from the hospital, he may not take his medications regularly. Why not? The reason may be simple. Perhaps no one took the time to tell him all he should know about his medication.

Avoid this problem. Instruct your patient carefully before he leaves the hospital. Choose a quiet time and place to talk to him. Use words he can understand. (If your patient's a child, use the same technique to instruct his parents.) Here are some guidelines:
• Make sure your patient knows the names of his medications and what each one is for. Ask him to repeat this essential information back to you.
• Tell him what good effects he may expect from his medication and what adverse effects he may have. Warn him to report adverse effects to the doctor but don't *overemphasize* them. You may discourage him from taking his medication.
• Stress the special considerations that pertain to his medication. For example, if he's taking a liquid medication that stains the teeth, such as hydrochloric acid, remind him to drink it through a straw and follow it with water.
• Tell him which foods, if any, will affect his medications and whether or not to take his medications with meals. Stress the importance of taking each medication at the proper time. If appropriate, warn him not to mix his medication with alcohol or other drugs.
• Don't expect him to stick to the hospital's routine when he goes home. Help him work out an acceptable schedule that's convenient for him.
• Tell him what to do if he misses a dose for any reason. For example, should he double his dose the next time? Or should he continue with the regular schedule?
• Avoid language that's confusing or misleading. For instance, don't say, "One tablet three times daily." Instead, be specific; say, "Take one tablet with breakfast, one with lunch, and one with dinner. Do this every day until all your tablets are gone."
• Be alert for personal problems that may prevent your patient from following your directions. For example, suppose he can't read well enough to understand the medication labels. Help him by making two large medication clocks like those shown on page 34.
• If his medication tastes unpleasant, share the tips listed on page 29 for making it more palatable.
• Remind him to take his medication for as long as ordered. If he stops taking it when his symptoms disappear, his condition may recur.
• Ask the patient to repeat your directions, so you're sure he understands them. Then, write them down so he, a family member, or a visiting nurse can refer to them at home. Make sure your handwriting's legible. You may find it helpful to give him a home care aid for each of his medications, like the one on the opposite page. Or give him an Identa-Drug Wallet™, as shown on the right.

Remember, some medications, such as steroids or hormones, are conveniently packaged according to dosage schedule. A plastic box with compartments, such as those made to hold sewing notions or fishing lures, may help the patient organize his schedule. Try one.

## Using an Identa-Drug Wallet™

Is your patient taking several different drugs? The Identa-Drug Wallet may help him keep them straight. First, fill in the ID card with your patient's name, address, age, and medical history. Slip it into the sleeve at the front of the wallet. Then, complete a drug card for each of the patient's drugs and put it in a drug card compartment. The manufacturer offers preprinted cards for 250 common drugs, and blank cards for drugs prescribed less frequently.

Finally, put a sample capsule or tablet into the pill well next to each card. Caution the patient that the samples are for reference only and shouldn't be swallowed. Now your patient has a handy reminder of what each drug looks like, what it's for, how and when to take it, and what side effects may accompany it.

To order an Identa-Drug Wallet and drug cards, write Cardiac Treatment Centers, Suite 211, Medical Arts Building, 890 Poplar Church Road, Camp Hill, Pennsylvania 17011.

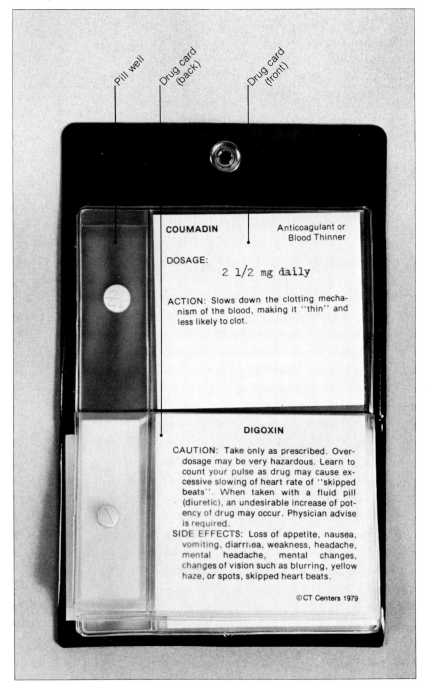

Pill well   Drug card (back)   Drug card (front)

**COUMADIN**    Anticoagulant or Blood Thinner

DOSAGE:

2 1/2 mg daily

ACTION: Slows down the clotting mechanism of the blood, making it "thin" and less likely to clot.

**DIGOXIN**

CAUTION: Take only as prescribed. Overdosage may be very hazardous. Learn to count your pulse as drug may cause excessive slowing of heart rate of "skipped beats". When taken with a fluid pill (diuretic), an undesirable increase of potency of drug may occur. Physician advise is required.
SIDE EFFECTS: Loss of appetite, nausea, vomiting, diarrhea, weakness, headache, mental headache, mental changes, changes of vision such as blurring, yellow haze, or spots, skipped heart beats.

©CT Centers 1979

# Patient teaching

# Home care

## Your medication:
## What you should know

Dear Patient:
The medication you're taking is _____
_____ .

The doctor has prescribed it because _____
_____ .

Take this medication exactly as the label directs.
Pay particular attention to these directions:
_____
_____ .

Avoid these foods or liquids while you're taking
this medication:
_____ .

But tell the doctor at once if you notice:
_____ .

Store your medication as follows:
_____ .

Important: Whenever you take any medication,
remember these guidelines:
• Follow the directions for taking medication
exactly. Don't try to make it last longer than the
doctor intended.
• Try to take your medication at the same time
each day. You'll be less likely to forget it.
• Don't permit others to take your medication,
and don't try any of theirs. The doctor's prescription is intended for your specific needs.
• If your medication is a liquid, use a measuring
spoon to ensure an accurate dose. Don't use a
regular eating spoon.
• Periodically, check the expiration date on the
label of your medication. Throw away any outdated medication, as well as medication that's
more than several years old.

# Home care

## Taking your medication

Dear Patient:
Your doctor has ordered the following medication
for you: _____
_____
_____
_____

The medication will help treat your: _____
_____
_____
_____
_____

Take the medication at these times: _____
_____
_____
_____
_____

Follow these instructions: _____
_____
_____
_____
_____
_____
_____
_____

Call the doctor if you notice any of the following:
_____
_____
_____
_____

# Oral administration

**How to make a medication clock**

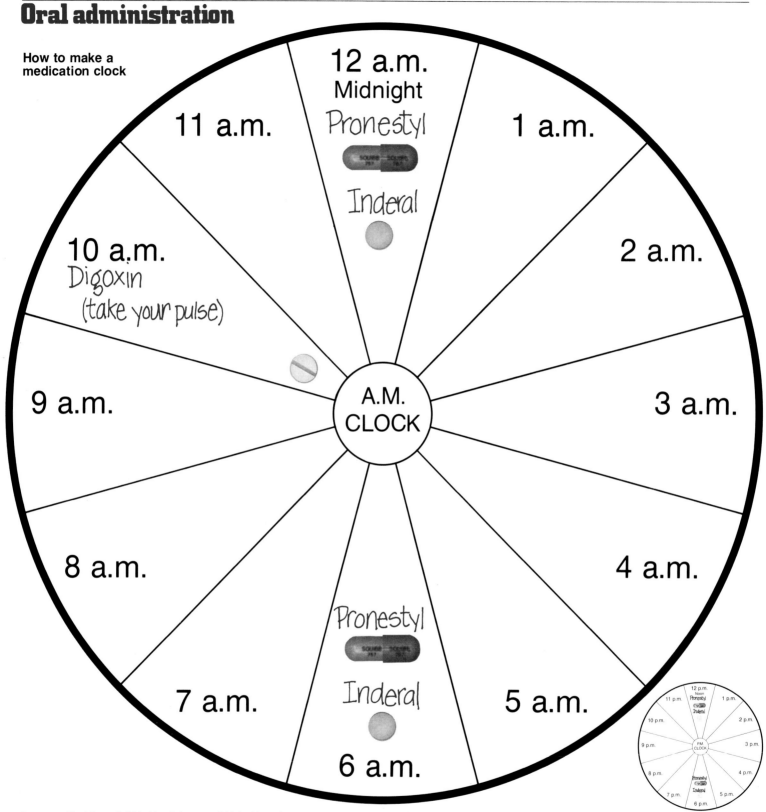

Is your patient forgetful? Is his vision poor? Help him take his medication on schedule by making two medication clocks like the ones shown here. Besides being easy to read and understand, these clocks will give your patient a sense of control over his own care. As a result, he'll be more likely to stick to his schedule.

Here's how to make the clocks. Just draw two large clock faces, each one a different color. Mark one A.M. and the other P.M. Make sure the numbers and letters are large and easy to read. Then, write in the names of your patient's medications beside the appropriate hours. If the medications are in tablet or capsule form, tape samples next to the names to remind him how each medication looks.

Tell the patient to take his clocks with him every time he visits the doctor. This way the nurse can update them if his medication schedule is adjusted. *Important:* Make sure your patient has a wristwatch or a clock that works. Remember, an elderly patient on a fixed income may not have the money to repair a broken timepiece.

PATIENT TEACHING

## Helping the elderly patient

Mr. Rossi, one of your elderly patients, is ready to go home after hospital treatment for cardiac disease. As you help him dress, you notice he seems preoccupied. When you ask what's wrong, he confesses, "I'm worried about all the medicine I'll have to give myself at home. The doctor says I need these pills to feel better. But I'm so forgetful these days. How will I keep them all straight?"

An elderly patient like Mr. Rossi may want to comply with his doctor's orders. But no matter how hard he tries to cooperate, his age may cause him problems.

How can you help? By making compliance as easy as you can for Mr. Rossi. Give him the same instructions you'd give any patient who's about to go home. (Review the checklist on page 32.) If possible, give instructions to a family member as well, because Mr. Rossi may need help at home. Now, here are some additional guidelines:
• Make sure the elderly patient can open his medication bottles easily. If he has arthritis or Parkinson's disease, he may not be able to remove a childproof cap. Get standard caps for all his bottles. Then, tell him to ask the pharmacist for standard caps whenever he needs refills.
• Tactfully inquire about his financial situation. If he's on a fixed income, he may not have the money to get his prescriptions refilled, as needed. So, to make his medication last longer, he may take less than the doctor ordered. Stress the importance of following the doctor's orders exactly. Then, refer him to your hospital's social service office for help.
• Ask about his eating habits. The doctor may want him to take some medications with meals. But if he habitually skips meals, he may miss one or more doses a day. Work out a realistic medication schedule, taking his eating habits into consideration. Then, contact a social service program, like Meals on Wheels, to help him to begin eating properly.
• Ask him to read his medication labels aloud. He may be embarrassed to admit that he can't see well enough. However, if he can identify his medications by color, ask the pharmacist to package them in clear bottles.
• If any of his medications must be packaged in an amber bottle to protect it from light, tape the medication label on the outside of the bottle. This way, the instructions won't be obscured by the tinted glass.
• If he has only two medication bottles, wrap a rubber band around one of them. Make sure he understands which of his bottles has the rubber band around it. Now, he can identify them by touch alone.
• Print the dosage instructions and schedule on a separate sheet of paper (using large letters), so your patient, a family member, or a visiting nurse can refer to them. Tape a sample tablet or capsule at the appropriate spot on the schedule, for reference. If you prefer, give him an Identa-Drug Wallet™ (see page 32). Or make him two large medication clocks, like the ones on the opposite page.
• Refer the patient to a rehabilitation program (if appropriate), as well as your community's Visiting Nurse Association, for follow-up.

## Giving medication by the sublingual or buccal routes

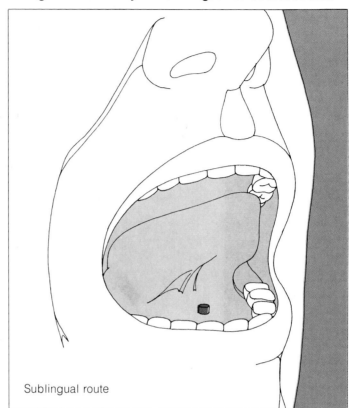

Sublingual route

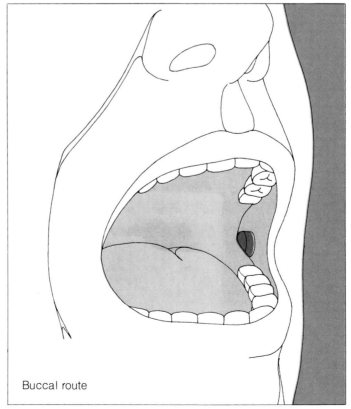

Buccal route

As you know, most oral medications are swallowed and then absorbed in the lower gastrointestinal tract. But a few—nitroglycerin and some male hormones, for example—may be absorbed directly into the circulation through the mucosa under the tongue (sublingual) or through the cheek mucosa (buccal).

Drug absorption via the mouth mucosa offers several advantages. For example, it permits direct entry of medication into the patient's bloodstream, so the medication takes effect quickly. In addition, it bypasses both the lower GI tract and the portal system, so the medication isn't transformed in the stomach, small intestine, or liver. And finally, the mucosa's convenient and safe to use.

To give tablets via this route, follow these instructions:
• *Sublingual:* Place tablet under the patient's tongue, as shown above. Ask him to hold it in place until it's absorbed.
• *Buccal:* Place tablet between the patient's cheek and teeth, as shown to the left. Ask him to close his mouth and hold the tablet against his cheek until it's absorbed.

In either case, caution the patient not to swallow the tablet. Then watch him closely as the medication's being absorbed.

# Tube administration

Chances are, you'll never use a gastric or nasogastric tube just to give medications. But if you use a tube to feed your patient, you can use it to give him oral medications, too.

Suppose your patient's recovering from neck surgery and has a nasogastric tube in place. Before you can safely give him medication, you must know if the tube's properly placed, and what to do if it's not. That's why, in this section, you'll see how to insert a nasogastric tube, and how to confirm proper placement. Then, you can administer medication through a nasogastric tube safely and confidently.

But what if your patient needs long-term or permanent tube feeding? Then the doctor may perform a gastrostomy. By suturing a gastric tube into the incision, he'll spare the patient repeated nasogastric tube insertions. Do you know how to give medication through a gastric tube? Can you change the dressing and care for the stoma site? And what if the tube becomes clogged or blocked? Do you know how to troubleshoot the problem? Read this section for the answers.

## Getting acquainted with tubes

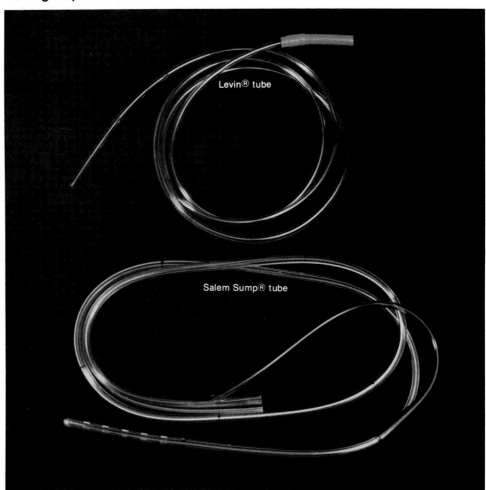

**1** Here are two common nasogastric tubes: the Salem Sump® and the Levin®. The radiopaque Salem Sump is really a tube within a tube. The smaller secondary tube permits continuous airflow for greater control of suction force. You can use the Y-port at the top of the tube to irrigate the patient's stomach.

Unlike the Salem Sump, the Levin tube is a single-lumen tube and is not radiopaque.

However, both tubes have multiple drainage openings, or eyes, on the bottom end. In addition, both have graduated markings to help you measure the correct length for insertion.

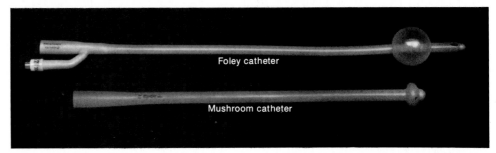

**2** If your patient has a gastrostomy, he probably has a Foley or a mushroom catheter sutured into his stoma. When inflated, the Foley's balloon holds the catheter securely in place, which is especially important if the sutures loosen. The mushroom catheter's bulb serves the same purpose. Like nasogastric tubes, both these catheters have eyes at the bottom end; however, neither is radiopaque.

## How to insert a nasogastric tube

**1** *If your patient's recovering from head or neck surgery, she may have a nasogastric tube in place for feeding. If she doesn't, you'll have to insert one before you can give oral medication. If this procedure's a nursing responsibility in your hospital, here's what to do:*

Begin by washing your hands and gathering the equipment in this photo. What size nasogastric tube do you need? Follow these guidelines: For an infant, obtain sizes 6 to 8 French; for an older child, sizes 8 to 12 French; and for an adult, sizes 12 to 18 French. When you've selected a tube, test its patency by running water through it. Examine it for roughness or ragged edges.

*Nursing tip:* Because most nasogastric tubes are made of vinyl plastic these days, the one you choose may be too stiff to insert gently. If it is, increase its flexibility by dipping it in warm water for several minutes. However, suppose you're using an older type rubber tube that's too pliant to maneuver easily during insertion. Remedy this by chilling the tube with ice.

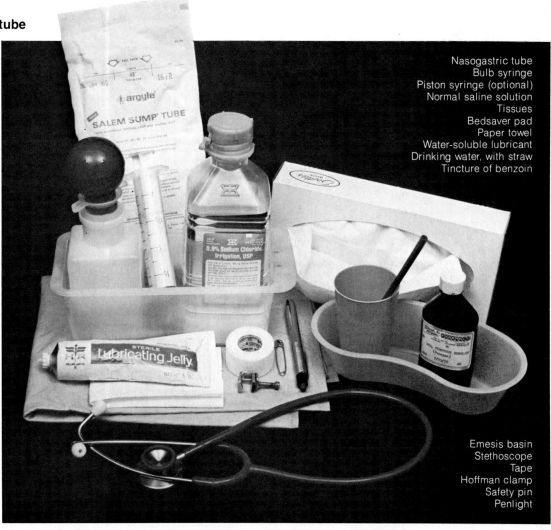

Nasogastric tube
Bulb syringe
Piston syringe (optional)
Normal saline solution
Tissues
Bedsaver pad
Paper towel
Water-soluble lubricant
Drinking water, with straw
Tincture of benzoin

Emesis basin
Stethoscope
Tape
Hoffman clamp
Safety pin
Penlight

**2** Next, tell the patient what you're about to do in words she can understand. Answer any questions she may have. To give her a sense of control during this uncomfortable procedure, agree on a signal she can use to tell you to wait for a moment; for example, raising her hand or tapping your arm. Then, place her in a comfortable upright position—either sitting or in a high Fowler's position. Protect her gown and the bed from spills by using bedsaver pads and a towel. Give her plenty of tissues, since intubation may stimulate tearing. Hand her the emesis basin in case she vomits.

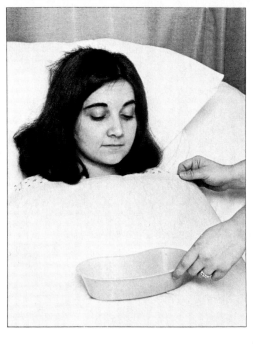

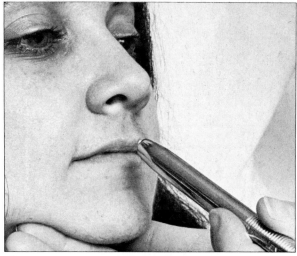

**3** Now, use a penlight to check her nostrils for possible obstruction. Then, alternately press each of her nostrils shut, and ask her to inhale through the open nostril. Choose the more patent of the two nostrils for insertion. (If neither is patent, notify the doctor.)

# Tube administration

### How to insert a nasogastric tube continued

**4** Use this simple two-step method to determine how much tube to insert. First, measure the distance from the patient's earlobe to the bridge of her nose, as shown here.

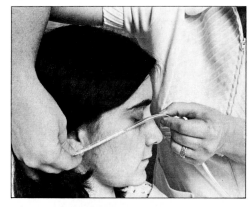

**5** Then, measure from the bridge of her nose to the bottom of her xiphoid process. Total these figures, and mark the desired length on the tube with adhesive tape.

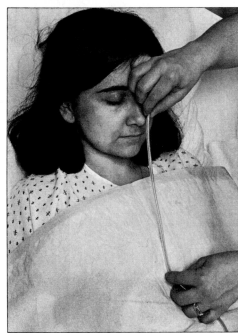

**6** If your patient's an infant or a child, measure him as follows: Turn his head to one side. Then, measure the distance from the tip of his nose to his earlobe; then from his earlobe to a point midway between the xiphoid process and the umbilicus. Total these measurements, and mark the tube.

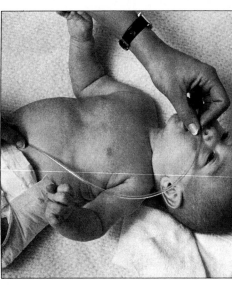

**7** When the tube's marked, hold it 6" to 8" (15.2 to 20.3 cm) from the tip. Roll it between your fingers to find its natural curve. If necessary, shape a curve yourself by tightly coiling the first 5" (12.7 cm) around your fingers, as shown here.

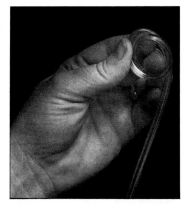

**8** Lubricate the first 6" (15.2 cm) of the tube with water-soluble lubricant. *Important:* Never lubricate a nasogastric tube with an oily lubricant like petroleum jelly. The patient may aspirate it and develop lipoid pneumonia.

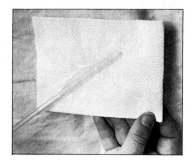

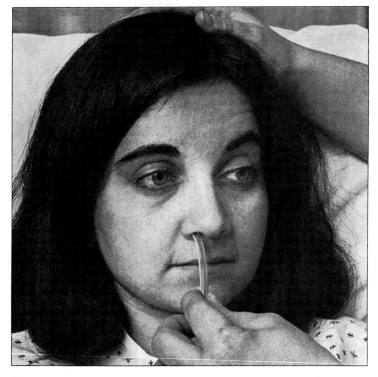

**9** Now you're ready to begin insertion. Ask the patient to hold her head upright, in a normal position. Then, insert the tube in the nostril you selected earlier. Following the tube's natural curve, gently advance it along the floor of the nasal passage. To make insertion easier, direct the tube toward the patient's ear on that side, *not* her other nostril.

**10** As the tip approaches her nasopharynx, rotate the tube 180° inward, toward the other nostril. Continue to advance it gently, until it's in the nasopharynx, pointing toward the esophagus. *Important:* Work slowly. If you feel resistance at any point, stop at once and withdraw the tube. Then, relubricate it and try the other nostril.

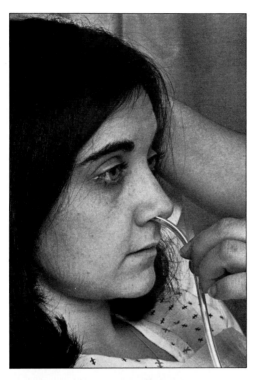

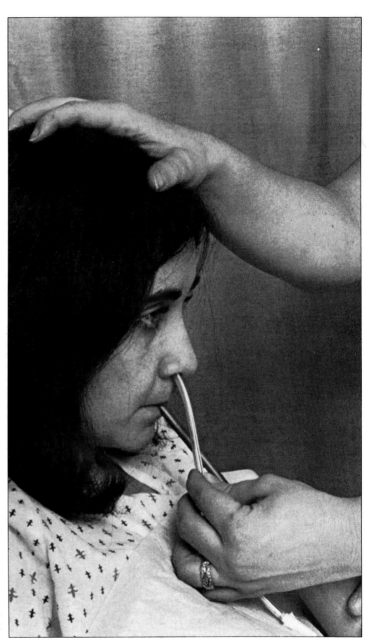

**11** As the tubing enters the patient's nasopharynx, she may gag. To prevent vomiting, stop advancing the tube, and tell the patient to take several deep breaths. Or ask her to take short sips of water through a straw. Either action will relax the pharynx and calm the gag reflex. In addition, the water will lubricate the tube.

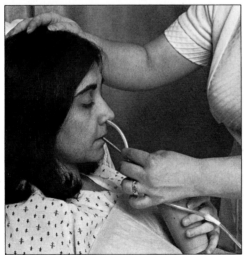

**12** Allow the patient a short rest. If she continues to gag, examine her throat. The tubing may be coiled there. If it is, withdraw it until it's straight.

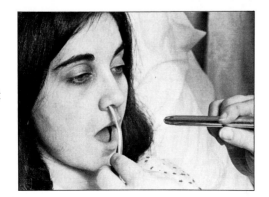

**13** When the patient's calm again, ask her to drop her head forward. This position will close her trachea and open her esophagus. Slowly advance the tubing into the esophagus.

To keep the patient from gagging, ask her to sip water while you advance the tube all the way to her stomach. Or ask her to chew ice chips throughout the procedure. Advance the tubing 3" to 5" (7.6 to 12.7 cm) each time she swallows.

🖙 *Nursing tip:* If she isn't permitted to drink water, ask her to dry-swallow at your signal.

Continue the process until the tube's inserted to the correct length. If you *can't* insert it that far, you may have inserted the tube in the patient's trachea, not her esophagus. Other indications that the tube may be in her trachea are vapor in the tubing and respiratory distress. Withdraw the tubing at once.

# Tube administration

### How to insert a nasogastric tube continued

**14** Even if the patient shows no sign of respiratory distress, make sure the tube's in her stomach, not a lung, before you proceed. Use at least two of the tests described below to verify proper placement. If *any* test suggests the tube's in the trachea or a lung, withdraw the tube at once and try again. Then, *always* reconfirm placement just before administering any fluids.

Here's the first test. When the tube's inserted, attempt to aspirate gastric fluid with a bulb or a piston syringe. You should be able to aspirate fluid easily, unless the tube's pressed against the stomach wall. If you have trouble, withdraw the tube slightly and try again. If you *still* can't aspirate gastric fluid, the tube's probably in a lung.

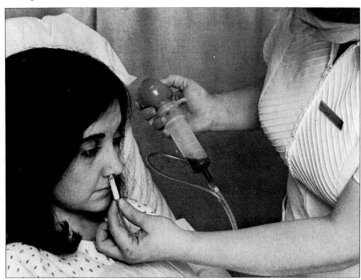

**15** Have you successfully aspirated stomach contents? Then flush the tube with 30 ml normal saline solution to clear gastric fluid from the eyes of the tube. Next, try a second test. Place a stethoscope over the patient's stomach, attach the syringe to the tube, and inject about 15 cc of air. If you hear a swooshing sound, air has entered her stomach. Silence indicates that the air's been absorbed by lung tissue.

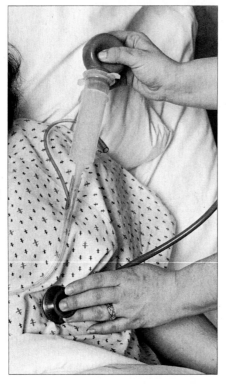

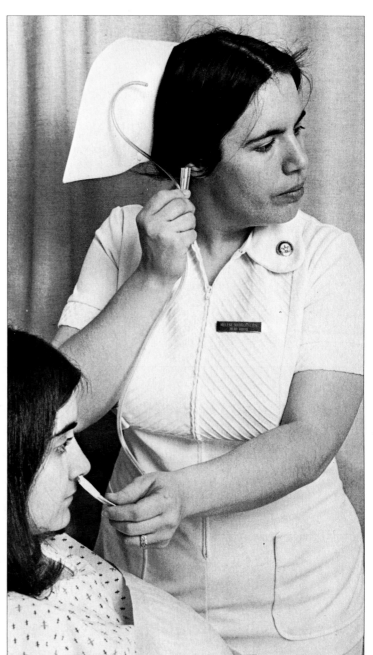

**16** The two tests shown on the left are probably the most reliable ways to confirm proper placement. But here are two alternate methods you may use.

Hold the end of the tubing to your ear, as the nurse is doing here. Listen closely. If the tube's in the patient's stomach, you'll hear nothing. But if it's in a lung, you'll hear crackling noises.

Or ask the patient to hum. If she can't, the tube's probably entered her trachea and separated her vocal cords.

*Note:* Some nurses place the end of the tube in a glass of water and watch for air bubbles as the patient exhales. But we don't recommend this method. It's dangerous, as well as unreliable. If the tube's in the patient's lung, she could aspirate water when she inhales.

**17** When you're sure the tube's correctly placed in the stomach, secure it with hypoallergenic tape. To do so, try this effective method: Crisscross a 2" strip around the tubing, just below her nose, and tape the ends to the top of the nose. Never tape the tube to the patient's forehead; positioning the tube this way may create a pressure sore inside the patient's nostril.

*Nursing tip:* If the tape won't stick to the patient's nose, apply tincture of benzoin first. Then, when the benzoin feels tacky, apply the tape over it

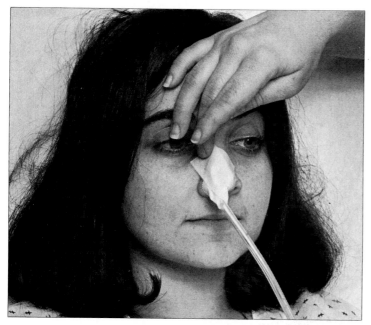

**18** After taping, plug the end of the tubing, or clamp it with a Hoffman clamp, as shown here. Cover the open end of the tube with gauze, to keep it clean. But if the patient complains of nausea, leave the tube unclamped until the feeling subsides. This will provide an opening for possible vomitus.

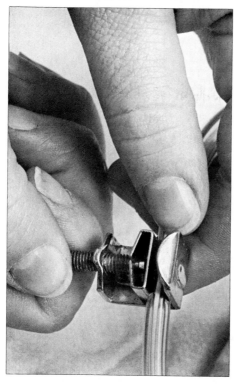

**19** To prevent the tube from dragging downward, wrap another piece of adhesive tape around the end of it and leave a tab. Then, safety-pin the tape tab to the patient's gown, just below shoulder level.

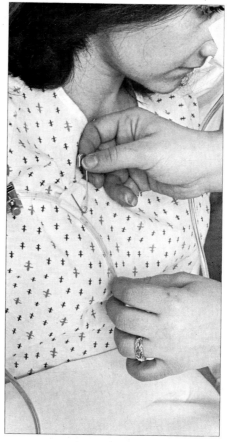

**20** As an alternative, loop a rubber band around the tubing in slipknot fashion. Then, pin the rubber band to the patient's gown, as shown in the inset.

Finally, document the entire procedure. Then, to make your patient as comfortable as possible, provide good mouth and nose care. Encourage her to brush her teeth regularly. Minimize nasal irritation by placing a small amount of water-soluble lubricant in each nostril. Prevent pressure sores by checking the patient regularly to make sure the tubing's positioned comfortably.

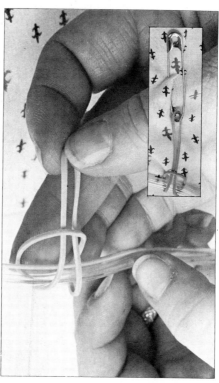

# Tube administration

### Giving medication through a nasogastric tube

**1** *You're about to give medication to a patient through a nasogastric tube. Before you begin, double-check the order, using the Five Rights system, and review any special considerations for the medication. For example, should you give it with tube feedings? If so, should you avoid giving certain foods at the same time? Remember, the action of oral medication doesn't change just because you're using a nasogastric tube. Make sure you know all the answers before you proceed. Then, follow these steps:*

First, measure the medication, and let it warm to room temperature. Remember, all medication given through a nasogastric tube must be in liquid form. Then, gather the equipment shown in this photo. If you prefer not to use a bulb syringe, substitute a small funnel or a 50 cc piston syringe.

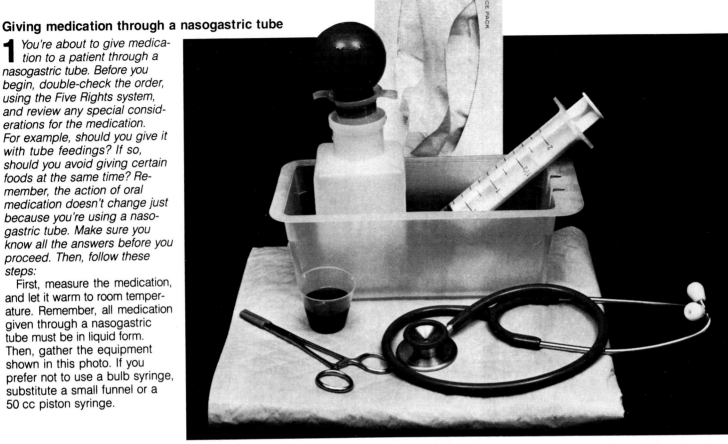

**2** After checking the medication order again, help the patient sit up. Remove the Hoffman clamp or plug from her nasogastric tube. Then, using at least two of the tests described on page 40, make sure the tube's properly placed in her stomach. Protect the patient's gown with a bedsaver pad or a towel, and give her tissues, in case she salivates excessively during the procedure.

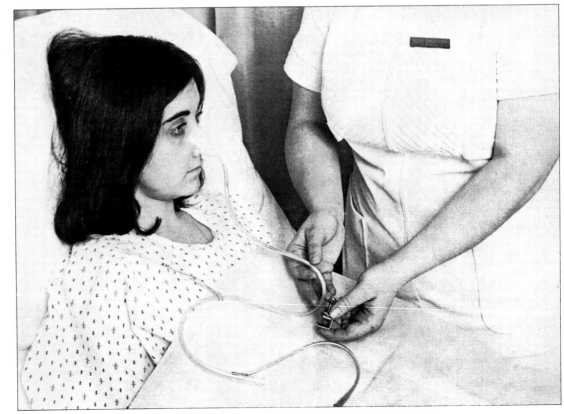

**3** Next, clamp the tube with a hemostat or by pinching it between your fingers. Remove the bulb or piston from the syringe (unless you're using a funnel), and attach the syringe to the tube, as shown here.

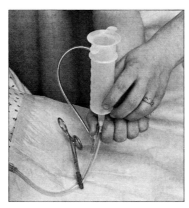

**4** Now, pour the medication into the syringe. Unclamp or release the tubing, and let the medication flow through it by gravity. *Never force liquids down a nasogastric tube.*

*Important:* Throughout the entire procedure, watch your patient's reactions. Stop the procedure immediately if she shows signs of discomfort. To control the flow of liquid, raise or lower the syringe height, or pinch and release the tube.

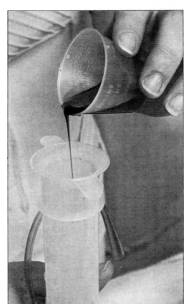

**5** Before the syringe empties completely, begin flushing the tube with 30 to 50 ml water. (If your patient's a child, use only 20 to 25 ml water.)

If you don't flush the tube, much of the medication will remain on the tube's sides and will never reach the patient. Flushing also clears medication from the eyes at the end of the tube, thereby reducing the chance of clogging.

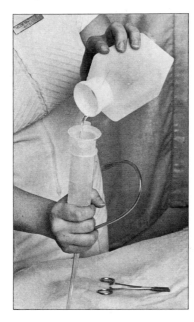

**6** After you've administered all the medication and water, remove the syringe (or funnel), and clamp or plug the tube. However, if your patient complains of nausea, leave the tube open until the feeling subsides.

Then, ask the patient to remain sitting in bed for approximately 30 minutes.

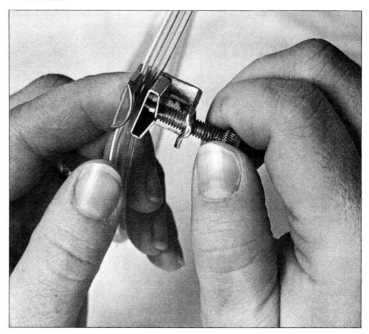

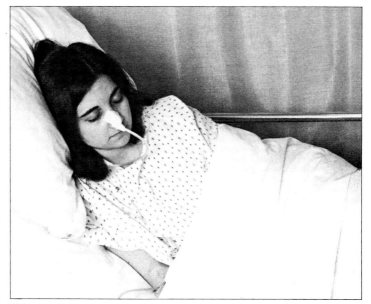

**7** If she's uncomfortable sitting, position her on her right side, with the head of the bed partially elevated. Either position will encourage her stomach to empty and discourage regurgitation.

📧 *Nursing tip:* A few medications, like antacids, should stay in the patient's stomach longer. To discourage gastric emptying, position the patient on her *left* side, with the head of the bed slightly elevated.

Finally, document the entire procedure in your nurses' notes.

# Tube administration

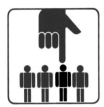

**When you give medication through a tube**

Whenever you give your patient medication through a gastric or a nasogastric tube, follow the same general procedure you learned for measuring and giving oral medications. Don't neglect all the special nursing considerations for the medication you're giving; for example, whether or not to give it with meals.

Also, remember these guidelines:
• Give medication in liquid form only. If the prescribed medication is a tablet or capsule (and can be crushed or opened), mix it with juice, water, or another compatible liquid. Remember, the drug particles must be small enough to pass easily through the eyes of the tube. Thoroughly mix the medication and liquid *before*

pouring them into the syringe. (For guidelines on crushing and opening solid medications, turn to page 22.)
• Dilute any viscous liquid medication with water or another liquid, unless contraindicated or incompatible, *before* putting them in the syringe.
• Avoid giving an oily medication. It'll cling to the sides of the tube and resist mixing with the flush solution.
• If you're giving the medication with a meal, give all the medication first. Why? Because if the patient can't tolerate an entire feeding, you may have to stop the procedure before he receives the medication.
• Never give an adult more than 400 ml liquid at a time. Never give an infant more than 120 ml liquid at a time.

## Removing a nasogastric tube

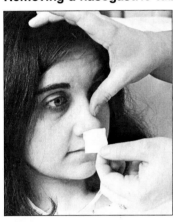

**1** *To remove a nasogastric tube correctly, follow these steps:* Ask the patient to sit upright, or place her in a high Fowler's position. Protect her gown with a towel or bedsaver pad. Release the tube that's pinned to her gown, and untape it from her nose.

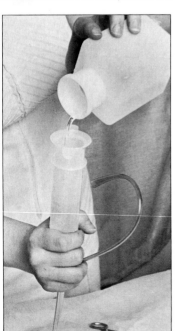

**2** Now, gently rotate the tube to make sure it moves freely. If it doesn't, try flushing the tube. To do this, remove the bulb from a bulb syringe, and attach the syringe to the tube. Pour 30 ml normal saline solution into the syringe, and unclamp the tube. Let gravity pull the solution down the tube. If the solution doesn't flow down the tube, try irrigating the tube very gently. But never irrigate forcefully.

If the tube still won't move freely, notify the doctor.

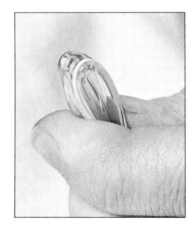

**3** When you're sure the tube's OK, get ready to withdraw it. Ask the patient to take—and hold—a deep breath. Reclamp the nasogastric tube with a hemostat, or fold it in your hand, as shown here. This will prevent any fluid in the tube from running down the patient's throat and getting into her lungs during withdrawal.

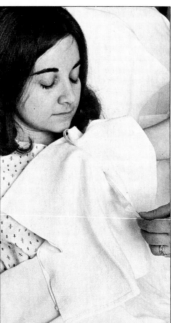

**4** Then, slowly withdraw the tube onto a towel, out of the patient's sight, if possible. When you're finished, tell the patient to resume breathing. Finally, document the entire procedure.

## Giving medication through a gastrostomy tube

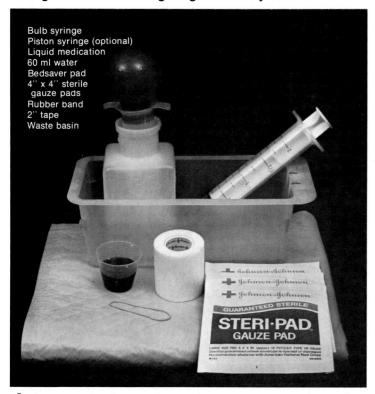

Bulb syringe
Piston syringe (optional)
Liquid medication
60 ml water
Bedsaver pad
4" x 4" sterile
 gauze pads
Rubber band
2" tape
Waste basin

**1** *Are you caring for a patient who's undergone a gastrostomy? Most likely, he has a Foley or a mushroom catheter in place. Here's how to give him medication.*

First, gather the equipment shown in this photo. (However, if you prefer, use a funnel instead of a syringe.) Make sure the medication's in liquid form and at room temperature. For guidelines on how to dissolve solid medications, see page 22.

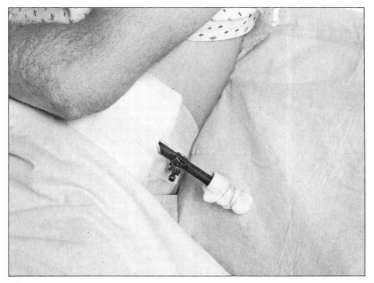

**2** After you've double-checked the order, using the Five Rights system, help the patient to a sitting or high Fowler's position. Protect the bed with a towel or bedsaver pad, and expose the gastrostomy site.

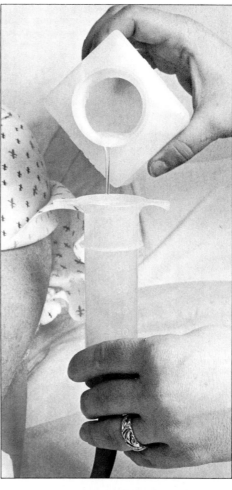

**3** Uncap the tube or unclamp it. Then, remove the bulb from a bulb syringe, and attach the syringe to the tube. Test the tube for patency by pouring about 30 ml water into the syringe. Let gravity carry the water into the patient's stomach.

If the tube's *not* patent, it may be pressed against the stomach wall. Try to free it by gently twisting it between your fingers. For other troubleshooting tips, turn to page 47.

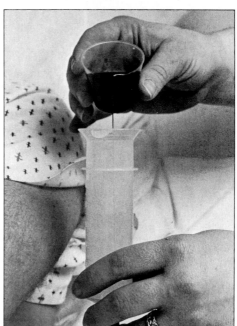

**4** Next, pour the correct amount of liquid medication into the syringe. Allow the medication to flow in gradually, by gravity. *Important:* If medication backs up in the tube or oozes around the suture line, stop the procedure at once, and notify the doctor.

# Tube administration

### Giving medication through a gastrostomy tube continued

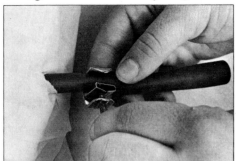

**5** Follow the medication with about 30 ml water, to clear the tube. Remove the syringe, and replace the tube's cap or clamp.

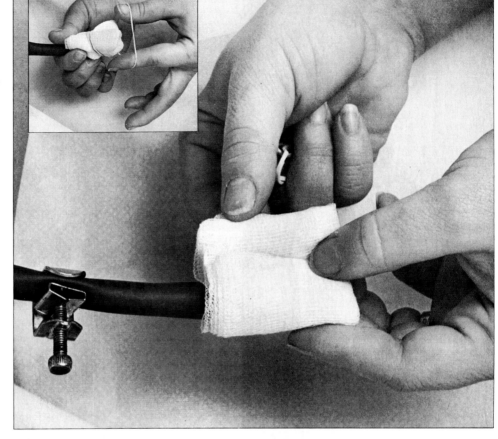

**6** When that's done, wrap a 4" x 4" sterile gauze pad around the open end to keep it clean (see the photo to the right). Then, secure the gauze with a rubber band, as shown in the inset.

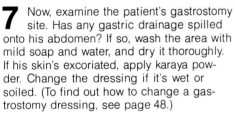

**7** Now, examine the patient's gastrostomy site. Has any gastric drainage spilled onto his abdomen? If so, wash the area with mild soap and water, and dry it thoroughly. If his skin's excoriated, apply karaya powder. Change the dressing if it's wet or soiled. (To find out how to change a gastrostomy dressing, see page 48.)

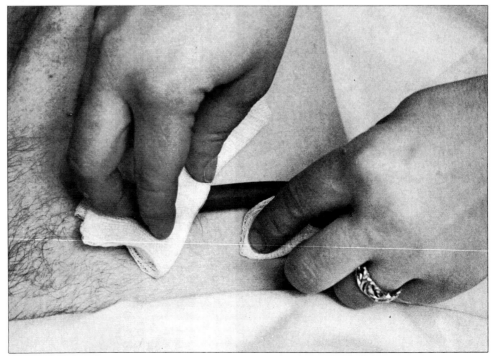

## When the gastric tube's not patent: How to irrigate

**1** *You're just beginning to pour water into your patient's gastric tube when it backs up in the tube instead of flowing into his stomach. Obviously, the tube's not patent, so you immediately stop the flow of water. What else should you do? First, try these tips. But if they don't help you solve the problem quickly, notify the doctor.*

If the tube isn't sutured in place, either internally or externally, gently twist it between your fingers, as shown here. If the tube is sutured in place, try repositioning the patient. If the tube's tip is pressed against the stomach wall, these movements may free it.

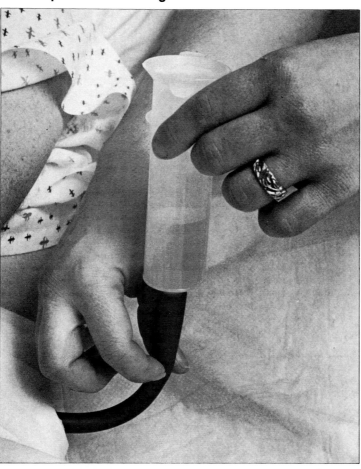

**2** If that doesn't work, compress the bulb and attach it to the syringe. Then, withdraw the water from the gastric tube. Remove the syringe and expel the water into a container (see inset). Then, reattach the syringe to the tube and try aspirating stomach contents. Caution: Never aspirate forcefully. If the tip of the tube's pressed against the stomach wall, vigorous aspiration may cause superficial erosion of the gastric mucosa.

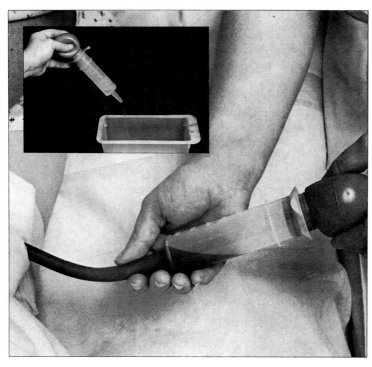

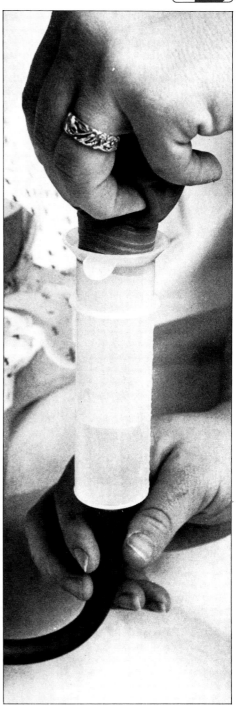

**3** Suppose this method doesn't work. If hospital policy permits, add 30 ml of water to the syringe. Compress the bulb firmly to push the fluid through the tube. Then, gently withdraw the fluid.

If you still have difficulty, use the syringe to inject 20 cc of air into the tube. Then, try aspirating again. If the tube's still not patent, notify the doctor.

# Tube administration

## How to change a gastrostomy dressing

**1** *If the dressing around your patient's gastrostomy tube becomes wet or soiled, will you know how to replace it? If not, study these photos.*

First, obtain some precut drainage sponges. If your hospital doesn't have any, make them yourself. To do this, simply hold two wrapped 4" x 4" gauze pads together, like this, and cut a slit halfway through the middle.

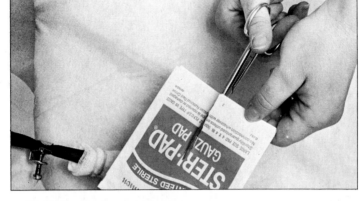

**2** Next, examine the skin around the patient's gastrostomy site. Is it clean and dry? If not, wash it with mild soap and water. Then, rinse and dry it thoroughly.

📧 *Nursing tip:* If the tube isn't held firmly in place by the sutures, tape it to the patient's abdomen, chevron style.

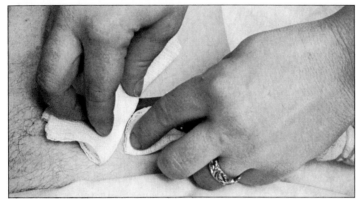

**3** Take the two 4" x 4" gauze pads out of their wrappers, and fit them snugly around the tube so the slit sides overlap.

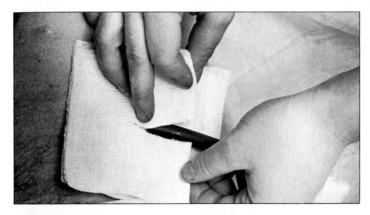

**4** Now, place an uncut 4" x 4" gauze pad directly on top of the two slit pads. Secure it with two strips of 2" tape.

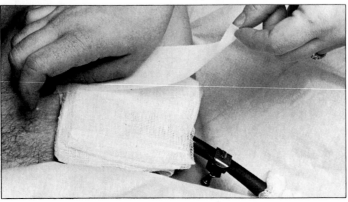

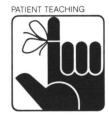

PATIENT TEACHING

**Teaching your patient gastrostomy care**

As soon as your patient is able to care for his gastrostomy himself, show him how. But remember, he'll probably need some extra support from you. Most likely, he'll have a hard time accepting the change in his body image and the loss of normal eating habits. But you can help him adjust by giving him control over his own care.

When you administer food or medication, or change his dressing, explain the procedure to him in words he can understand. Encourage him to ask questions. Then, make sure you're nearby the first few times he tries each procedure himself, in case he needs help or encouragement. Then, when he's ready for discharge, give him a copy of the home care aid on the opposite page.

# Patient teaching

# Home care
## How to care for your gastrostomy

Dear Patient:

Your doctor has placed a tube in the opening to your stomach. The nurse has shown you how to use it. Here are some guidelines to help you when you return home.
• For your comfort, make sure any fluids entering your stomach are warmed to room temperature.
• To feed or medicate yourself, sit down and attach a clean funnel or syringe (with the plunger or bulb removed) to the tube. Then, unclamp the tube.
• Make sure the tube's not clogged by pouring about 2 tablespoons (30 ml) water into the funnel. (If the water doesn't flow into your stomach, the tube's probably clogged. Stop the procedure, and call your doctor immediately.)
• When you're certain the tube's open, pour the food or medication into the funnel. Let it drip slowly into your stomach. Don't try to rush the procedure by forcing it.
• After the food or medication's completely in your stomach, clear the tube by pouring 2 more tablespoons of water into the funnel.
• Replace the clamp on the tube, and remove the funnel. (If you lose the clamp, fold the tube on top of itself and fasten it with a rubber band.)
• Cover the end of the tube with a gauze pad to keep it clean. Then, wrap a rubber band around the pad to hold it in place.
• Stay seated upright for at least 30 minutes after your meal.
• Using warm water, wash the funnel thoroughly after every use.
• Keep the skin around your stomach opening clean and dry. If it becomes irritated, dust it with karaya powder, as you were instructed in the hospital.
• Change your dressing once a day or whenever it becomes wet or soiled.
• Examine the skin around the opening. Call your doctor if the skin feels sore, looks red, or seems puffy. Also, call your doctor if you find food or medication seeping from the insertion site or if you feel any discomfort in your stomach.

# Rectal administration

Do you know why the doctor may choose the rectal route to give your patient medication? What special steps should you take before giving a retention enema? How do you insert a rectal suppository correctly, so the patient will get maximum benefit from the medication?

On the following pages, you'll learn about different types of rectal medications. What's more, you'll see exactly how to administer them. But keep in mind that a tactful, compassionate approach on your part is just as important as your skill in giving the medication. Do your best to preserve the patient's dignity throughout any rectal procedure. Assure privacy by closing doors and curtains completely. Avoid exposing him unnecessarily. Above all, provide continuous reassurance and support.

## Using the rectal route for systemic effects: Pros and cons

*The doctor may want you to give your patient medication by the rectal route, because it offers these advantages:*
• provides a safe route if your patient's vomiting, unconscious, or unable to swallow
• provides an effective route to treat vomiting
• doesn't irritate the patient's upper GI tract, as some oral medications do
• avoids destruction of medication by digestive enzymes in stomach and small intestine
• avoids biotransformation in liver, since drugs absorbed from the lower rectum bypass the portal system.

*However, the rectal route also has these disadvantages:*
• may be uncomfortable and embarrassing for the patient
• may result in irregular or incomplete drug absorption, depending on the patient's ability to retain the medication and whether or not feces are present in his rectum. Because rectal absorption may be incomplete, rectal dosages of some medications may be larger than oral doses.
• may stimulate the patient's vagal nerve by stretching his anal sphincters. For this reason, you must use the rectal route cautiously with cardiac patients.

## Nurses' guide to rectal medications

### Suppository

**Description**
A solid medication in a firm base, such as cocoa butter, that melts at body temperature. May be molded in a variety of cylindrical shapes. Usually about 1½" (4 cm) long (smaller for infants and children).

**Type for local use**
• Analgesics
• Astringents
• Antipruritics
• Anti-inflammatories
• Laxatives, lubricants, and cathartics
• Carminatives

**Type for systemic use**
• Analgesics
• Antiemetics
• Antipyretics
• Bronchodilators
• Sedatives
• Hypnotics

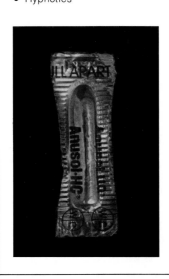

### Ointment

**Description**
A semisolid medication that may be applied externally to the anus, or internally to the rectum.

**Type for local use**
• Antipruritics
• Astringents
• Analgesics and anesthetics
• Anti-inflammatories
• Antiseptics

**Type for systemic use**
• None

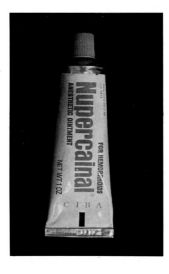

### Enema

**Description**
Liquid given as either a *retention* enema (retained by the patient for at least 30 minutes or until absorbed) or a *nonretention* enema (retained by the patient for at least 10 minutes and then expelled).
*Note:* Enemas given to cleanse the lower bowel aren't usually medicated.

**Type for local use**
• Anthelmintics
• Astringents
• Laxatives, lubricants, and cathartics
• Antiseptics
• Steroids

**Type for systemic use**
• Antipyretics
• Sedatives
• Anesthetics
• Nutritives and water

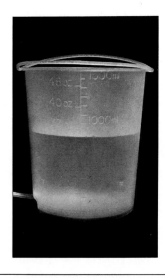

## Nurses' guide to enemas

Use this chart as a guide when you give your patient an enema. But before you decide which guidelines are appropriate, consider the type of medication the doctor has prescribed, as well as your patient's age, size, and condition. For instance, if your patient's a small 9-year-old child, use the smallest tube suggested for his age-group. Physical size is more important than age.

Always use smaller tubing and less solution when you give a retention enema. Why? Because this combination will create less pressure in the patient's rectum and make retention easier. *Note:* Never give a retention enema to an infant or young child. Neither will be able to retain it.

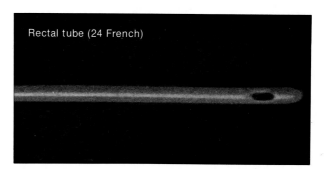
Rectal tube (24 French)

### Retention enemas

| Age-group | Rectal tube size | Amount of tube to insert | Amount of fluid to introduce |
|-----------|------------------|--------------------------|------------------------------|
| Adults | 14 to 20 French | 3'' to 4'' (7.5 to 10 cm) | 150 to 200 ml |
| Children over age 6 | 12 to 14 French | 2'' to 3'' (5 to 7.5 cm) | 75 to 150 ml |

### Nonretention enemas

| Age-group | Rectal tube size | Amount of tube to insert | Amount of fluid to introduce |
|-----------|------------------|--------------------------|------------------------------|
| Adults | 22 to 30 French | 3'' to 4'' (7.5 to 10 cm) | 750 to 1,000 ml |
| Children over age 6 | 14 to 18 French | 2'' to 3'' (5 to 7.5 cm) | 500 to 1,000 ml |
| Children over age 2 | 12 to 14 French | 1½'' to 2'' (3.75 to 5 cm) | 500 ml or less |
| Infants | 12 French | 1'' to 1½'' (2.5 to 3.75 cm) | 250 ml or less |

PATIENT PREPARATION

### Preparing to give a medicated retention enema

Giving a medicated retention enema requires good planning. For example, you must schedule the procedure before meals. Why? Because a full stomach triggers peristalsis, making retention more difficult for the patient.

Before beginning, you also must check your patient's condition. Notify the doctor if:
• your patient's constipated. Feces in his rectum will interfere with drug absorption. The doctor may want you to administer a cleansing nonretention enema first.
• the patient has diarrhea. In this case, the drug may be expelled before it can be absorbed. The doctor may

want you to check for a fecal impaction before he treats the diarrhea. Then, he may want to choose another route.
• the patient has an inflamed rectum. An enema may exacerbate the condition. The doctor may want to choose another route.

Always take enough time to thoroughly prepare the patient for the procedure. You'll need his cooperation. Make sure he understands the purpose of a retention enema and the importance of retaining the medication until it's absorbed. Finally, to reduce the risk of stimulating peristalsis during the procedure, ask him to empty his bladder and rectum before you begin.

# Rectal administration

## How to administer a retention enema

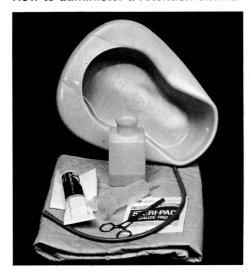

**1** *If you've prepared the patient for a retention enema, you're ready to begin the procedure. Wash your hands and remember to maintain clean technique. Then follow these steps:*

First, gather the equipment shown here: a pitcher or other small container to hold the enema solution, a bulb syringe (with bulb removed), a rectal tube or catheter, water-soluble lubricant, a bedsaver pad, a paper towel, 4" x 4" gauze pads or tissues, a bedpan, and a hemostat.

To avoid stimulating peristalsis when you give the enema, heat the solution to about 105° F. (40.6° C.) before administering it. Make sure the temperature's correct by testing it with a bath thermometer or pouring a little of the solution over the inside of your wrist.

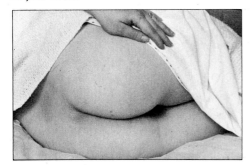

**2** Provide privacy for your patient by closing the door and pulling the bed curtain. Adjust the bed so it's flat. Then, position your patient on her left side, with her right knee flexed. This will permit the enema solution to flow naturally into the descending colon.

Is this position uncomfortable for your patient? Place her on her right side or back instead.

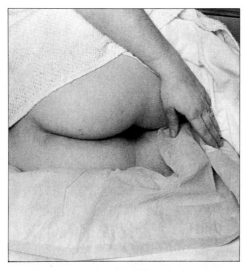

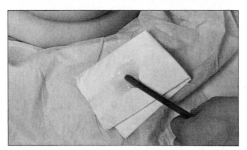

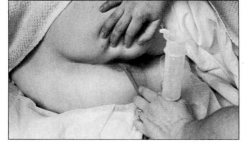

**3** To protect the bed linen, place the bedsaver pad under the patient's left buttock. Tuck part of the pad between her legs, as shown here, to catch any fluid that escapes from her rectum. Expose her anus, but provide a drape so she has some privacy. Reassure her, so she won't be unduly embarrassed.

**4** Flush air from the tube. To do this, first remove the bulb from the syringe, and attach the syringe to the tube. Next, double up the tube in one hand, and pour in a small amount of solution. Then, lower the open end of the tube. When the solution flows out the end, pinch the tube between your fingers, as shown here.

Once again, fold the tube in one hand. Then clamp it, as shown in the inset photo. Leave the syringe attached.

**5** Now, place a little water-soluble lubricant on a paper towel. Lubricate the tip of the tube by rolling it in the lubricant.

**6** With your free hand, separate the patient's buttocks, so you can see her anus. Ask the patient to breathe deeply through her mouth, to help relax her anal sphincters. With your other hand, gently insert the tube, and direct it toward the patient's umbilicus.

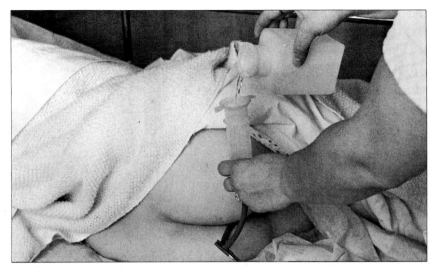

**7** Advance the tube about 4" (10 cm). Make sure it's past the internal anal sphincters or it may be expelled. *Important:* If you feel any resistance, withdraw the tube, and notify the doctor. Forcing it may damage the patient's mucous membranes.

Now, hold the syringe about 5" (12.7 cm) above her anus. Slowly pour the warmed solution from the container into the syringe, as shown here.

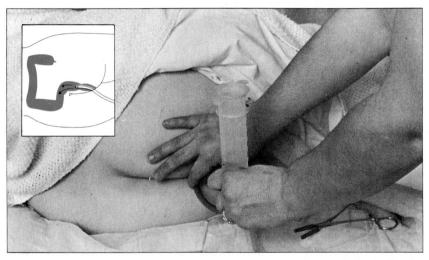

**8** Next, remove the clamp, and let the solution flow into patient by gravity (see inset). Don't try to rush the procedure by pouring the solution faster or raising the syringe height. By increasing fluid pressure in the rectum, either action could stimulate an urge to defecate. *Important:* Throughout the procedure, do your best to keep your patient comfortable. If she feels cramps or an urge to defecate, stop administering the enema immediately by pinching the tube. Tell the patient to breathe deeply, to help her relax. When she's comfortable again, proceed cautiously. Do everything possible to help her retain the enema.

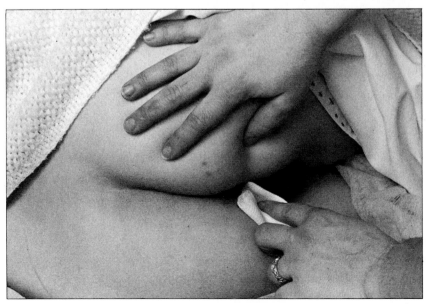

**9** As soon as you've administered all the enema solution, clamp the tubing, and ask the patient to take a deep breath. Then, withdraw the tube gently but quickly.

Hold the patient's buttocks together, or press firmly on her anus with a 4" x 4" gauze pad or tissue, until the urge to defecate passes. Then, wash and dry her buttocks. Remember to wash your hands after the procedure.

How long should the patient retain the enema? This'll vary according to the type of medication. As a rule, however, she should hold it for at least 30 minutes.

To make it easier for her, keep her as quiet and comfortable as possible. Leave the bedsaver pad in place, to guard against seepage, and put the bedpan within reach. Don't run water within the patient's hearing. If the patient still has trouble retaining the enema solution, try one of the suggestions shown on page 54.

After the prescribed length of time, tell the patient she may defecate. Then, document the procedure in your nurses' notes.

# Rectal administration

## Helping the patient retain an enema

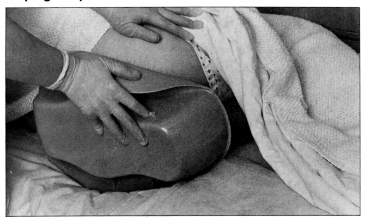

**1** *Are you caring for an elderly patient? She may have difficulty retaining an enema for any length of time.* So, before you begin the procedure, put on gloves to protect your hands if she expels the solution immediately. Then, place a bedpan under her left hip and against the buttock. Protect the bed linen with a bedsaver pad.

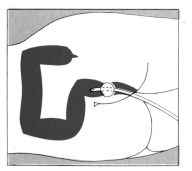

**2** If hospital policy permits, use a Foley catheter as a rectal tube. After you've inserted it, inflate the catheter's balloon with 5 to 10 ml water. Then, gently pull the catheter back against the internal anal sphincter. The balloon will seal off the patient's rectum.

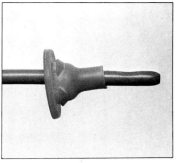

**3** Or try this suggestion to seal off the patient's rectum: Cut off the tip of a baby bottle nipple, and slip it over the end of a rectal tube, as shown here. Then, when you push the nipple snugly against the patient's anus, you'll find it forms a watertight seal.

## Administering a nonretention enema

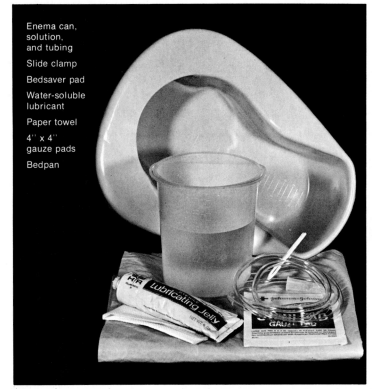

Enema can, solution, and tubing

Slide clamp

Bedsaver pad

Water-soluble lubricant

Paper towel

4'' x 4'' gauze pads

Bedpan

**1** *You've just learned how to give a retention enema. But suppose the doctor wants you to give a nonretention enema. Do you know how the procedures differ? If not, study this photostory.*

First, obtain a disposable enema kit. In addition to the equipment shown here, you'll need an I.V. pole.

If your hospital can't supply a disposable enema kit, gather the equipment you need. You may substitute an enema can and a rectal tube with an enema bag, but don't forget the clamp.

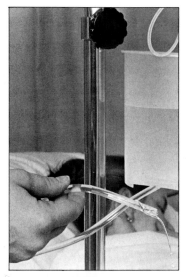

**2** Heat the solution to about 105° F. (40.6° C.), and pour it into the enema container. Now, hang the enema container 12'' to 18'' (30.5 to 46 cm) above the bed. Then, allow a small amount to flow through the tubing, to expel all the air. Clamp the tubing.

*Note:* If a female patient has a condition affecting her reproductive organs, hang the container *level* with her upper hip.

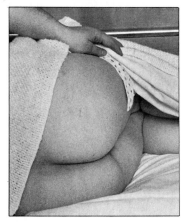

**3** Don't forget to close the door and the bed curtain to ensure privacy. Prepare and position the patient on her left side, as we explained on page 52.

**Administering a nonretention enema** continued

**4** Now, lubricate the tubing. Expose your patient's anus, and ask her to breathe deeply. Gently insert the tube about 4" (10 cm) into her rectum. Open the clamp slightly, and allow the enema solution to flow into the tube slowly. If the patient says she wants to defecate, or complains of cramps or a full feeling, stop the flow temporarily. Then, when she feels more comfortable, resume the flow until the container's *almost* empty.

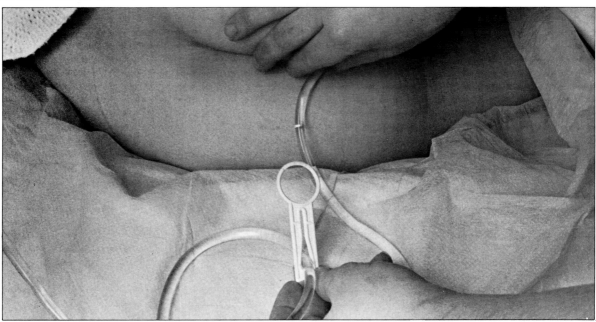

**5** Then, clamp and remove the tubing. *Important:* Don't let the container become completely empty before you clamp it or you may introduce air into the rectum.

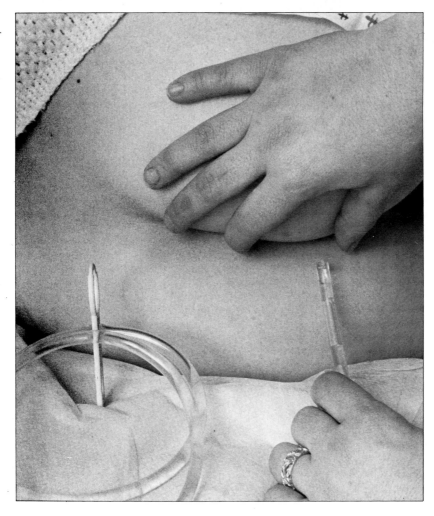

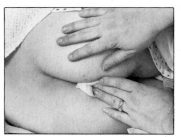

**6** When the tube's removed, hold the patient's buttocks together or press on her anus with a 4" x 4" gauze pad or tissue until her urge to defecate subsides. Keep the bedpan within her reach, but encourage her to retain the enema for at least 10 minutes before expelling it. (If the patient's unable to expel the enema within a reasonable period of time, you may have to siphon it out. To learn how, see page 56.)

Finally, wash and dry the patient's anal area, and ventilate her room. Use an air freshener, if necessary. Then, document the entire procedure, including the following information: type and amount of enema solution used; amount, color, and consistency of expelled feces; amount of flatus expelled; reduction in abdominal distention, if any; and patient's tolerance of the procedure.

# Rectal administration

## How to withdraw an enema

**1** *Suppose you gave your patient a nonretention enema more than 30 minutes ago and she still hasn't expelled it. What should you do?*

First, try this simple method to withdraw it. Turn the patient to her *right* side, as you see here. This position encourages her descending colon to empty (see inset).

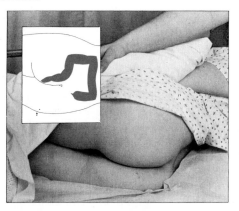

**2** Make sure the bed linen is protected with a bedsaver pad. Then, put a bedpan on a chair beside her bed, *below* the level of her rectum. Lubricate and insert a tube (size 22 to 30 French) into her rectum. Hold the other end of the tube over the bedpan. Gravity will help withdraw the enema.

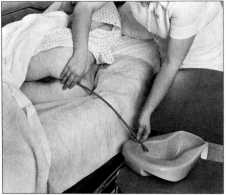

**3** What if this method doesn't work? You may have to *siphon* the enema. But check your hospital's policy about this first. In some hospitals, this procedure requires a doctor's order.

Here's how the siphoning procedure is done: Position the patient and the bedpan as explained above. Then, remove the bulb from a bulb syringe, and connect the syringe to the rectal tube, as shown here. (If you prefer, use a small funnel instead of a syringe.)

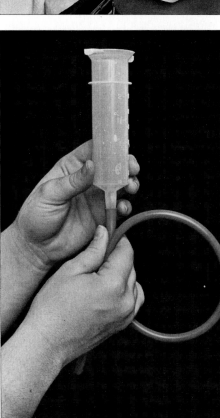

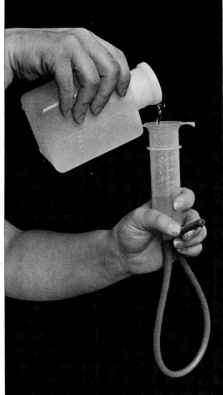

**4** Fill the syringe half full with warm tap water. Flush and clamp the tubing, as shown on page 52.

**5** Next, lubricate and insert the rectal tube about 4" (10 cm) into the patient's rectum. Holding the syringe above her anus, unclamp the tube to allow a small amount of water to flow into the patient.

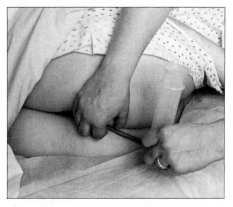

**6** Quickly lower and invert the syringe over the bedpan. Pressure and gravity will combine to pull the water from the patient's rectum.

Document the entire procedure. Include the amount, color, and consistency of the siphoned fluid and expelled feces (if any).

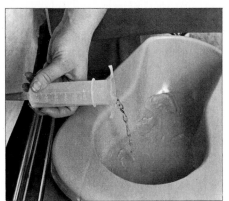

## How to insert a rectal suppository

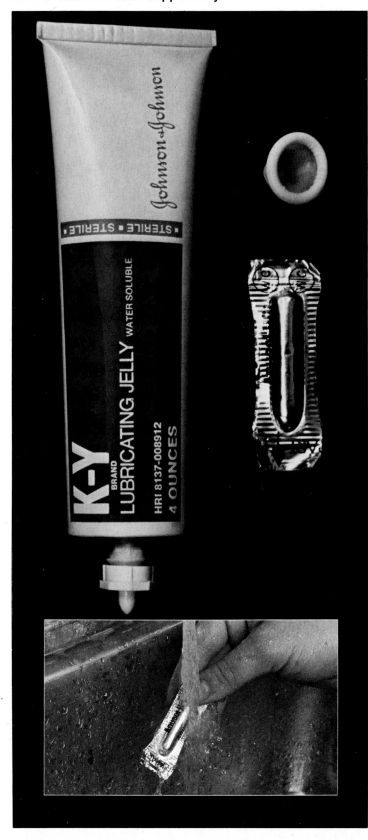

**1** *Has the doctor ordered a suppository for your patient? These photos will show you how to administer it.*

First, wash your hands and gather the equipment you'll need: the suppository, a glove or finger cot, and water-soluble lubricant.

*Nursing tip:* If the suppository's too soft, it'll adhere to the wrapper. As shown in the inset photo, remedy this by holding it under cold running water until it becomes firm. Or place it in the medication refrigerator for several minutes.

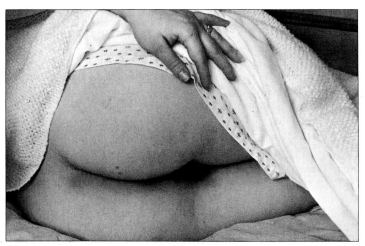

**2** Next, provide privacy for your patient by closing her door and drawing the bed curtains. Explain the procedure, and position her so her anus is exposed. (Choose any position that she finds comfortable.)

*Important:* Is your patient unconscious? Don't let this keep you from explaining the procedure. Remember, an unconscious patient may later recall everything you said. Your reassuring words will encourage her to relax.

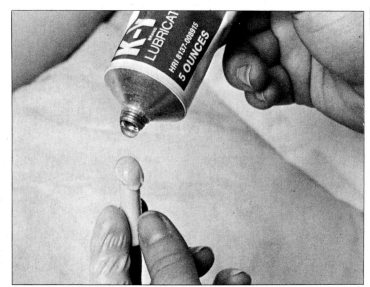

**3** After you've prepared the patient, you're ready to begin the procedure. Put on a glove or finger cot. Remove the suppository from the wrapper, and lubricate it with water-soluble lubricant.

# Rectal administration

**How to insert a rectal suppository** continued

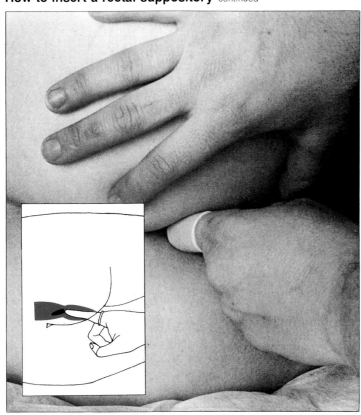

**4** With your ungloved hand, separate the patient's buttocks so you can see her anus. Ask her to take a deep breath. With your gloved hand, gently insert the suppository into her rectum, tapered end first. Use your forefinger to direct it along the rectal wall, toward the umbilicus. Continue to advance it 3" (7.5 cm), or about the length of your finger, until it's passed the patient's internal anal sphincter (see inset). Otherwise, it may be expelled. *Important:* Take care not to push the suppository into a fecal mass.

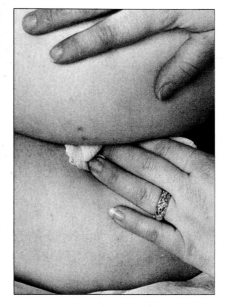

**5** Is the suppository in place? Hold the patient's buttocks together, or press on her anus with a 4" x 4" gauze pad or tissues until her urge to defecate subsides. Then, clean excess lubricant from the anus.

Urge the patient to retain the suppository for at least 20 minutes. Remove your glove or finger cot, wash your hands, and document the procedure. *Note:* If you gave the suppository to relieve constipation, tell your patient to defecate as soon as she feels an urge.

---

**Applying rectal ointments**

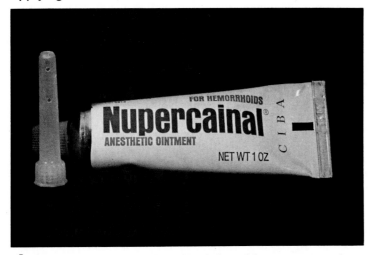

**1** *If your patient's rectum is sore or inflamed for any reason, she may need a rectal ointment applied, for its soothing local effect. To apply the ointment externally, wear gloves or use a gauze pad. But to apply it internally, use an applicator like the one shown in this photo.*

First, get the prescribed tube of ointment and a tapered applicator with openings along the sides. Also obtain water-soluble lubricant, a bedsaver pad, and several 4" x 4" gauze pads.

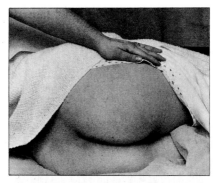

**2** Make sure you provide privacy for your patient, and explain what you're going to do. Then, place her on her side with the top leg flexed, so you can see her anus easily. (If she can't tolerate a side position, you may substitute one that's more comfortable for her.) Protect the bedding with a bedsaver pad.

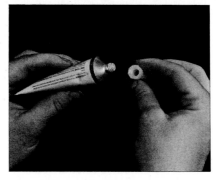

**3** Figure on using approximately 1" (2.5 cm) of ointment. To gauge how much pressure to use, try squeezing out the correct amount before you attach the tube to the applicator. Then, attach the applicator to the tube, as shown here, and coat the applicator with water-soluble lubricant.

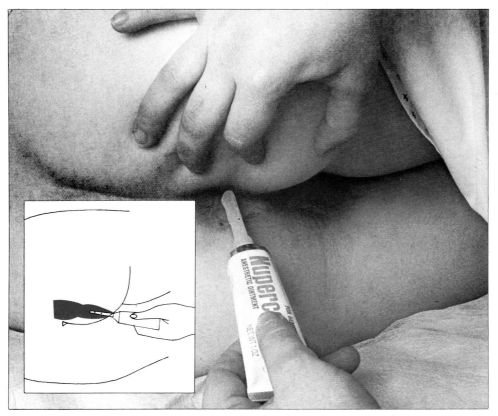

**4** Expose the patient's anus with one hand, and ask the patient to take several deep breaths through her mouth, to relax her anal sphincters.

[Inset] Then, slowly insert the applicator into her anus, directing it toward her umbilicus. Keep in mind that the patient's rectum is probably tender, so be gentle.

**5** When you've inserted the entire applicator, slowly squeeze the tube to eject the medication. Remove the applicator.

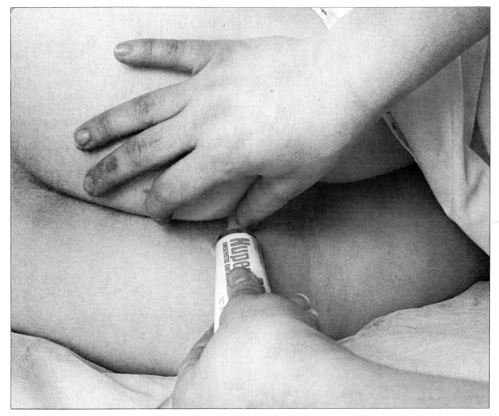

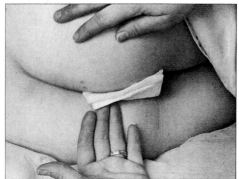

**6** Place a folded 4" x 4" gauze pad between the patient's buttocks to absorb excess ointment. Disassemble the tube and applicator, and recap the tube. Clean the applicator thoroughly with warm water and soap. Finally, document the procedure.

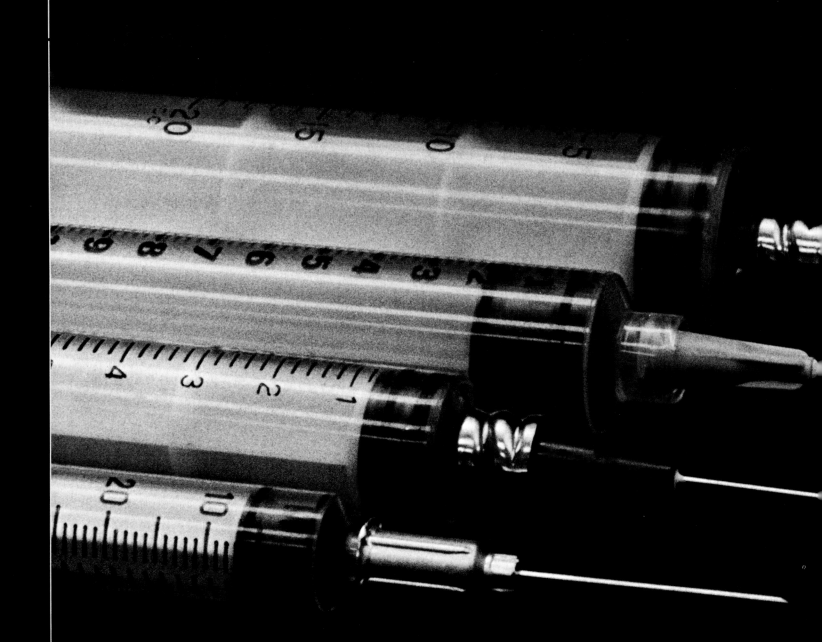

# Administering by the Parenteral Route

Parenteral administration
Intradermal administration
Subcutaneous administration
Intramuscular administration
Intravenous administration
Intra-arterial administration

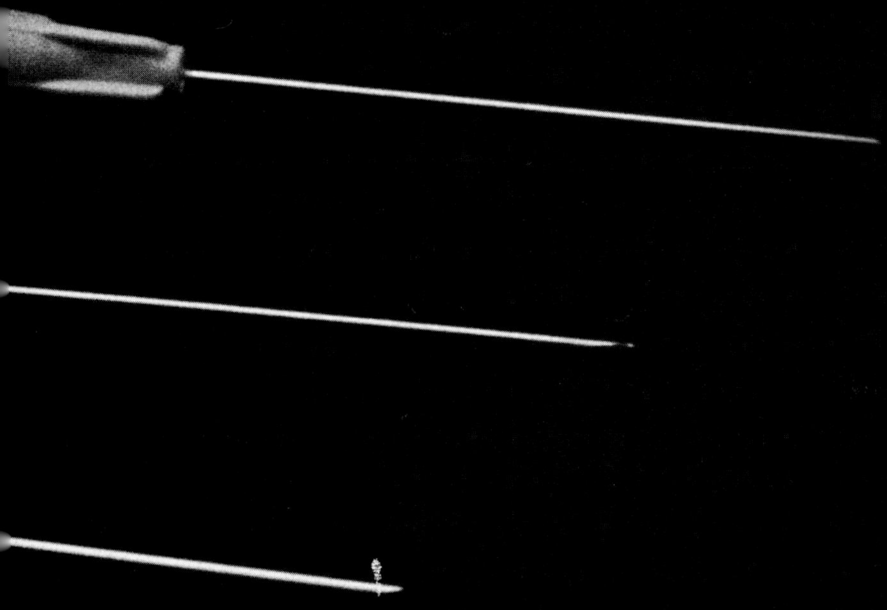

# Parenteral administration

Let's assume you're planning to use the parenteral route to give your patient his medication. Begin by familiarizing yourself with the few pieces of basic equipment you'll use: a syringe, a needle, the prescribed medication, and skin prep material.

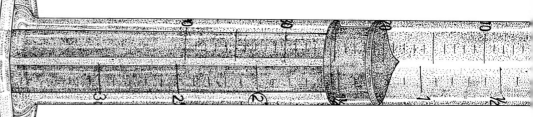

Then, read the rest of this section. We'll tell you what you need to know about injecting medication by each parenteral route.

### Nurses' guide to parenteral injection equipment

#### Syringes

Syringes are available in reusable glass or disposable plastic. Disposable plastic syringes are most widely used today. You've probably used a syringe many times. To alter the space within the syringe barrel, depress or pull back on the plunger. *Important:* When you handle the syringe, make sure you don't contaminate the plunger, the inside of the barrel, or the syringe tip. Maintaining sterility is an important part of giving injections.

#### Medications

The medication that's been ordered may be a liquid or a powder. Liquid medications may come in glass ampules or glass vials and are ready to draw into a syringe. To do this properly, follow these instructions:

If the medication comes in a vial, clean the stopper with alcohol. Pull back the syringe plunger until the amount of air in the barrel equals the exact amount of medication you want to withdraw from the vial. Then, insert the needle into the vial stopper, inject the air, and withdraw the medication.

If the liquid medication comes in a glass ampule, withdraw the medication this way: Score the neck of the ampule with a razor blade. Then, wrap it in a semidry alcohol swab. Grasp the ampule and snap off the top. Place the needle in the open ampule, and withdraw the prescribed dose.

If the medication you're going to inject comes in a powder, you'll have to reconstitute it. To do this, you'll need the medication, a vial of a compatible diluent, an 18G needle and syringe, and an alcohol swab.

After you've assembled the equipment, remove the protective cap from the diluent vial, and swab the stopper with alcohol. Then, follow the steps shown below:

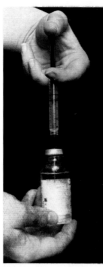

**1** Inject air equal to the recommended amount of diluent into the vial, as shown here.

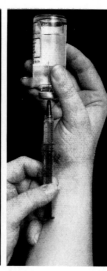

**2** Then, draw up the recommended amount of diluent into the needle and syringe.

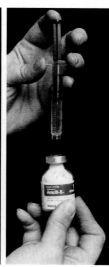

**3** Swab the medication bottle's stopper, and inject the diluent into the bottle.

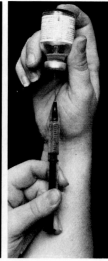

**4** Mix the medication and diluent; then draw up the reconstituted medication.

### Needles

Now examine the needle, which as you know must be kept sterile. You'll find that needles come in various lengths, diameters (called gauges), and bevel designs. The illustrations below will help you select the correct needle for the route you're using.

#### Intradermal

For an intradermal injection, select a needle ⅜" to ⅝" in length, 25G to 26G in diameter, with a short bevel.

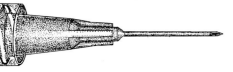

#### Subcutaneous

For a subcutaneous injection, select a needle ⅝" to ⅞" in length, 24G to 27G in diameter, with a medium bevel.

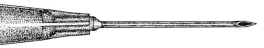

#### Intramuscular

For an intramuscular injection, select a needle 1" to 3" in length, 19G to 23G in diameter, with a medium bevel.

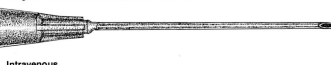

#### Intravenous

For an intravenous injection, select a needle 1" to 3" in length, 16G to 21G in diameter, with a long bevel.

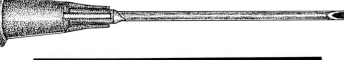

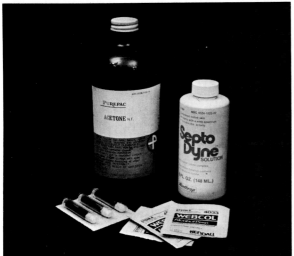

### Skin preps

Several types of skin preps are available, the most common being ethyl alcohol. All of them are applied in the same manner—working from the center of the site outward, in a circular motion; and all serve the same purpose—disinfecting the patient's skin.

## Injection tips

Of all the ways to give medications, injection is the most hazardous. If you inject a medication incorrectly, you may damage the patient's nerves, tissue, or blood vessels, or introduce bacteria into his system. To avoid complications, follow these guidelines:
- Select the site carefully to avoid major nerves and blood vessels.
- Don't select areas that have lesions, inflammation, hair, or birthmarks.
- Use only sterile needles and syringes.
- Make sure the needle you select is the proper length for the injection and the patient's body size.
- Always check for blood backflow before injecting. For intradermal, subcutaneous, and intramuscular injections, you don't want a backflow. If you notice blood in the syringe barrel, remove the needle and replace it with a new one. Then select another site and try again. (Be sure to discard both needles afterward.) For intravenous injections, you must get a blood backflow before proceeding. This tells you the needle's in the vein.
- Make sure someone's nearby to help restrain the patient, if necessary.
- Establish a site rotation plan for the patient who'll undergo repeated injections. Record the plan on his Kardex, so everyone can refer to it.

## When injections scare your patient: What to do

Is your patient terrified by the thought of a needle puncturing his skin? He's not alone. Many people fear injections, even though they may regard them as the most effective form of drug treatment.

What can you do about this fear? Master the techniques explained here for reassuring your patient. It's one of your greatest challenges.

### Talk to him first

Preparing your patient for an injection begins with finding out what he already knows. Ask him if he's ever had an injection. If he has, ask him what type it was; also, where on his body it was given. Then, inquire how he felt about it. He may confide that he finds injections frightening. Or he may tell you it was extremely painful.

Allow him plenty of time to talk. As you explain what kind of injection you're going to give, encourage his questions and answer them honestly. Try to correct any misconceptions he may have. Explain why the injection's important to his therapy and how it will help.

### Reassuring the child

Preparing a child for an injection doesn't vary much from the procedure explained above. However, you may find that he's more frightened than most adults and less able to understand the injection's importance.

To help, try to get acquainted with the child before the procedure. Then, when the time comes for it, tell him what you're going to do in words he can understand. Be honest. If he asks if it will hurt, tell him that it may, but explain that his cooperation will make it less painful.

Give the child as much control over the situation as possible. For example, let him choose which arm to inject. If that's not possible (for instance, if a specific rotation plan has already been designated), find another way to let him help.

If you must restrain him for the injection, enlist the help of someone other than a parent. Involving one or both parents may make him associate them with the pain of the injection. Instead, have them nearby (if possible), so they can comfort their child immediately afterward.

Don't expect a child to be stoic about the injection. Tell him it's OK to cry if he wants. Suppose he feels like punching something. Encourage him to use a pillow. You may even suggest that he give a play injection to a doll or a stuffed animal.

Put an adhesive bandage strip over the site if the child desires one. Such a bandage is unnecessary clinically, but it serves several other important functions: It makes the child feel protected; it allays his fear that blood will leak from the site; and it acts as a badge or an award.

# Intradermal administration

When was the last time you injected medication intradermally? If you're like most nurses, you probably don't perform an intradermal injection very often. That's why the next several pages are important. In them, you'll learn:
* the best injection sites

* the proper injection techniques
* how to read injection results
* the ins and outs of immunotherapy.
    You'll also learn special techniques and nursing tips that'll increase your self-confidence. Read on to brush up on your knowledge of intradermal injections.

**Nurses' guide to intradermal injection sites**

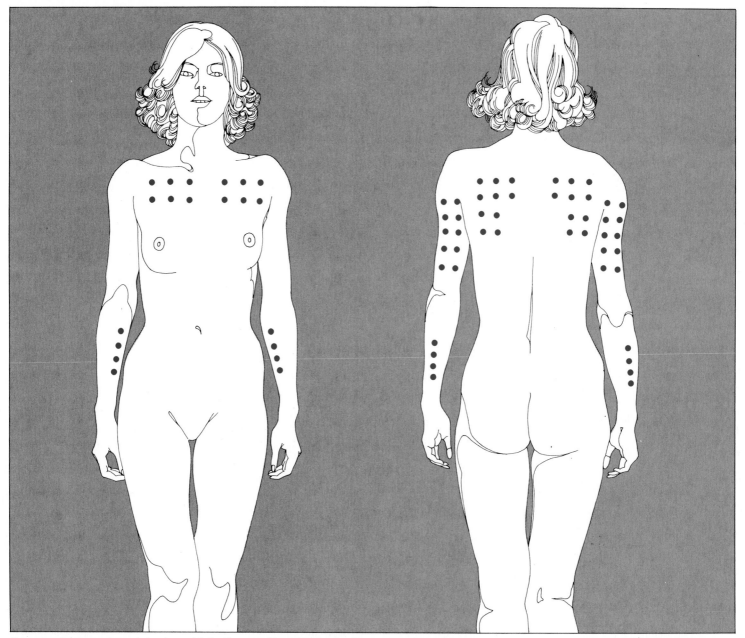

If your patient needs an intradermal injection, you'll probably give it in her ventral forearm. But if her arms are burned or irritated, you could substitute her upper chest or a shoulder blade. The sites you can use are shown here. The skin in these areas is lightly pig- mented, thinly keratinized, and usually hairless. These qualities make it easy to observe reactions to the injection. *Note:* Don't expect *immediate results*. The capillaries of the dermis have a slower absorption rate than subcutaneous tissue or muscle.

## Nurses' guide to diagnostic skin antigens

| Generic and trade names | Indications and dosage | Side effects | Nursing considerations |
|---|---|---|---|
| **histoplasmin\*** 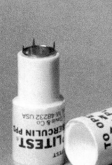 | *Suspected histoplasmosis*— **Adults and children:** 0.1 ml of 1:100 dilution intradermally on inner forearm. Use tuberculin syringe with 26G or 27G ⅜" needle. | *Local:* urticaria, ulceration or necrosis in highly sensitive patients *Other:* shortness of breath, sweating, anaphylaxis | • Read test at 24 to 48 hours. Induration of 5 mm or more is positive. • Reaction may be depressed in malnutrition or in immunosuppression. • Crossreaction may occur with other fungi (e.g., *Candida albicans, Blastomyces dermatitides*). • Obtain accurate history of allergies and past reactions to skin tests. • Keep epinephrine 1:1,000 available. • Cold packs or topical corticosteroids may relieve pain and itching if severe reaction occurs. |
| **Old tuberculin** Old Tuberculin Test\*; Tuberculin, Mono-Vacc Test; Tuberculin Tine Test | *Diagnosis of tuberculosis*— **Adults and children:** 10 tuberculin units (0.1 ml of 1:1,000) Old tuberculin intradermally on inner forearm. In suspected tuberculosis, use 1 tuberculin unit first. Use tuberculin syringe with 26G or 27G ⅜" needle. Multiple-puncture test: cleanse skin thoroughly with alcohol; make skin taut on inner forearm; press points firmly into selected site. | *Local:* hypersensitivity (vesication, ulceration, necrosis) *Other:* anaphylaxis | • Use cautiously in active tuberculosis. • False positive reaction can occur in sensitive patients. • Reaction may be depressed in malnutrition or in immunosuppression. • Read test in 48 to 72 hours. Induration of 10 mm or more is positive; 5 to 9 mm, doubtful; less than 5, negative. • Multiple-puncture test: 1 to 2 mm induration is positive. • Old Tuberculin Tine Test equals 5 tuberculin units purified protein derivatives. • Obtain accurate history of allergies, especially to acacia (contained in tine test as stabilizer), and past reactions to skin tests. • Keep epinephrine 1:1,000 available. • Subcutaneous injection invalidates test results. Bleb must form on skin upon injection. • Corticosteroids and other immunosuppressants may suppress skin test reaction. • Cold packs or topical corticosteroids may relieve pain and itching if severe reaction occurs. |
| **tuberculin purified protein derivative, Mantoux** Aplisol, Aplitest, Sclavo test-PPD, Sterneedle, Tuberculin PPD-Heaf, Tuberculin PPD-Stabilized\*, Tubersol\* | *Diagnosis of tuberculosis*— **Adults and children:** 5 tuberculin units (0.1 ml) intradermally on inner forearm. Suspected sensitivity dose is 1 tuberculin unit. Patients failing to react to 5 tuberculin units should be tested with 250 tuberculin units. First strength equals 1 tuberculin unit/0.1 ml; intermediate strength, 5 tuberculin units/0.1 ml: second strength, 250 tuberculin units/0.1 ml. Use tuberculin syringe with 26G or 27G ⅜" needle. Multiple-puncture test: cleanse skin thoroughly with alcohol; make skin taut on inner forearm; press points firmly into selected site. | *Local:* pain, pruritus, ulceration, necrosis *Other:* anaphylaxis | • Contraindicated in known tuberculin-positive reactors; severe reactions may occur. Use cautiously with active tuberculosis. • Read test in 48 to 72 hours. Induration of 10 mm or more is positive; 5 to 9 mm, doubtful; less than 5 mm, negative. • Multiple-puncture test: vesication is positive reaction; induration of less than 2 mm without vesication is negative. • 1 tuberculin unit may give false negative test; 250 tuberculin units may give false positive test. • Obtain accurate history of allergies and past reactions to skin tests. • Reaction may be depressed in malnutrition, immunosuppression, or viral infections (up to 4 weeks postinfection). • Solution adsorbed by plastic. Use at once after drawing into plastic syringe. • Keep epinephrine 1:1,000 available. • Subcutaneous injection invalidates test results. Bleb must form on skin upon injection. • Cold packs or topical corticosteroids may relieve pain and itching if severe reaction occurs. • Never give initial test with second test strength (250 tuberculin units). • A tine test is available for rapid screening. • Corticosteroids and other immunosuppressants may suppress skin test reaction. |

\*Available in the United States and in Canada.

# Intradermal administration

### Injecting intradermally

**1** *You're caring for 47-year-old Matt Hiller who has a respiratory infection that the doctor suspects is histoplasmosis. To determine the exact diagnosis, the doctor orders a histoplasmosis skin test.*

*You know the histoplasmosis bacteria has to be injected intradermally, but do you know how? This photostory will show you.*

Begin by assembling your equipment. You'll need the medication, a 1 cc tuberculin syringe, a 26G ⅝" needle, acetone, a 4" x 4" sterile gauze pad, and several alcohol swabs. If your patient has a history of allergic reactions to drugs, like Mr. Hiller, you'll also need normal saline solu-tion or an allergy test diluent, plus another needle and syringe. You'll use this extra equipment to make a control wheal.

Attach the needles to the syringes. Check the medication to make sure it's not out-dated or contaminated. If the medication's OK, draw it up into one of the syringes. Then, cap the syringe and bring all the equipment to the patient's bedside.

Tell him what you're going to do. Position him with his ventral forearm exposed and supported on a flat surface, and his elbow flexed. Whether the patient's sitting or lying down makes no difference. Just make sure he's comfortable.

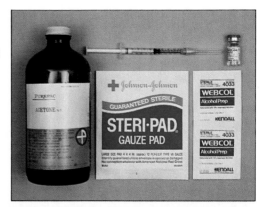

**2** Next, locate his antecubital space. Then, measure several finger-widths away from it in the direction of the hand. You should end up about a handbreadth away from the wrist. Avoid any area covered with hair or blemishes. These could make reading the test results difficult.

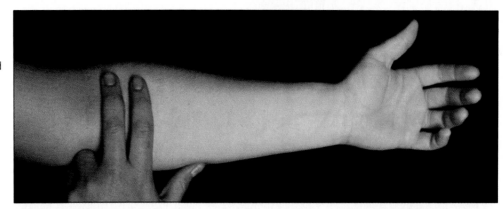

**3** Defat the skin with acetone, by begin-ning at the center of the site and moving outward, in a circular motion. Then, prep the skin with an alcohol swab follow-ing the same method. Never use a disinfec-tant like Betadine, which will discolor the skin. And don't rub so hard you cause irritation. Either action could hinder the reading of the test.

Allow the skin to dry thoroughly. If you inject the patient while the skin's wet, you may accidentally introduce antiseptic into the dermis.

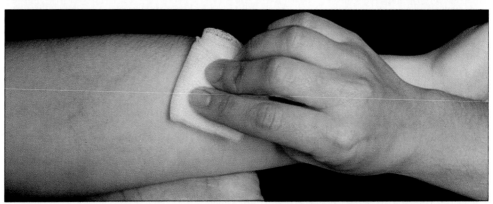

**4** Hold the patient's forearm in one hand, and stretch his skin with your thumb, as shown here. Then, with your other hand, hold the syringe between your thumb and forefinger, and rest the plunger against the heel of your palm. Expel any air in the needle.

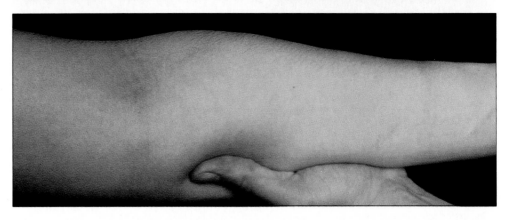

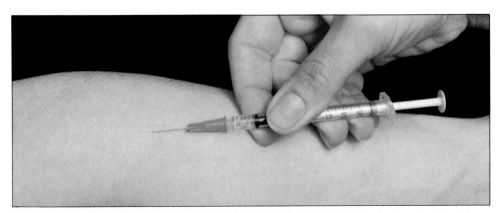

**5** Position the syringe so that the needle is almost flat against the patient's skin. Make sure that the bevel of the needle is up.

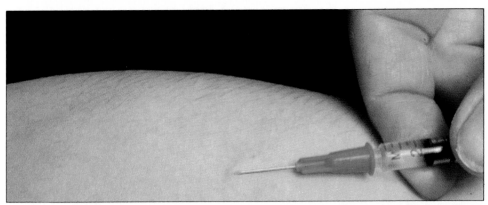

**6** Insert the needle by pressing it against the skin until you meet resistance. Then, advance the needle through the epidermis, so that the point of the needle is visible through the skin. Stop when it's resting ⅛" (3 mm) below the skin's surface, between the epidermis and the dermal layers.

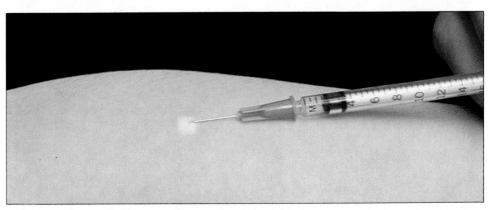

**7** Now, inject the medication as slowly and gently as possible. Expect to feel some resistance, which is your assurance that the needle's properly placed. If the needle moves freely, you've inserted it too deeply. Withdraw it slightly and try again. When you've finished injecting the medication, leave the needle in place momentarily. Watch for a small white blister or wheal to form, about 6 mm in diameter.

*Important:* If you're injecting test doses of penicillin or tetanus antitoxin, be alert for signs of anaphylaxis.

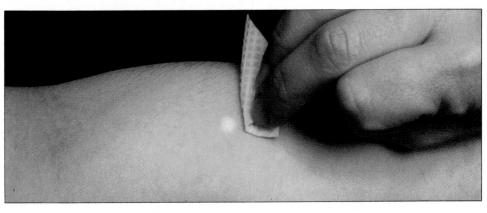

**8** When the wheal appears, withdraw the needle, and apply gentle pressure to the site. Don't massage it, because doing so may interfere with test results.

Now, make a control wheal. Draw up normal saline solution or allergy test diluent in the second syringe. Inject it into the opposite arm, using the same procedure.

Document the name of the medication and the amount given. If the patient has an allergic reaction to the injection within 30 minutes, notify the doctor. In most cases, a reaction occurs within 48 to 72 hours. For guidelines on how to read it, study the illustration on the following page.

# Intradermal administration

## Reading a diagnostic skin test

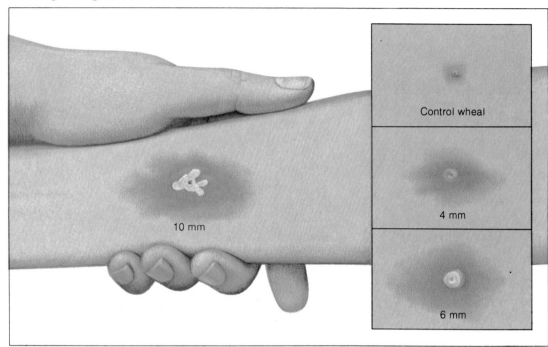

Control wheal

10 mm

4 mm

6 mm

The area around the injection site should be hard before you begin your reading. Record the extent of induration in millimeters. Also measure erythema if it's present. But remember, erythema without hardening is not significant.

Suppose you're testing for tuberculosis. Use the test result scale shown to the left to measure the extent of induration. But keep in mind that different tests have different scales. Check the package insert that comes with the medication first.

Examine the site. If the indurated area is less than 5 mm in diameter, consider the test result negative. If it's 5 to 9 mm in diameter, consider the result doubtful and perform another test. If it's 10 mm or more, the result is positive. Your patient may have tuberculosis. The doctor will order treatment.

## Learning about immunotherapy

Immunotherapy remains a relatively unconventional way to treat cancer, but it may be more widely used in the future. When immunotherapy is administered, it's usually in addition to surgery, radiation therapy, or conventional forms of chemotherapy.

Here's how immunotherapy works: Scientists tell us that the body produces cancer cells all the time. But the body's immune system usually combats these malignant cells successfully and prevents tumors from developing. Immunotherapy is the injection of an agent (such as BCG, C Parvum, or MER) that stimulates and aids the body's natural responses to cancer. Before you administer immunotherapy, learn its advantages and disadvantages.

**Advantages**
• The medication doesn't cause cell destruction, unlike other forms of cancer treatment.

• The medication aids and stimulates the body's normal cancer defenses, instead of introducing toxic substances.
• Side effects are fewer and milder than those with other forms of cancer treatment.

**Disadvantages**
• Patient may experience malaise, flu-like syndrome, low-grade fever, chills, and less commonly, nausea and vomiting.
• Patient may suffer from jaundice and, in rare cases, tuberculosis.
• Patient's hepatic function tests may show abnormalities.
• Patient may experience lymph node swelling, pain, and localized abscesses and drainage near the injection site.
• Skin may become inflamed and ulcerated if injection site isn't rotated.

If you're instructed to perform immunotherapy, you'll inject one of these three bacterial preparations:

| Preparation | Description | Administration |
|---|---|---|
| **BCG** (bacillus Calmette-Guérin) | Attenuated form of the tubercle bacillus | Directly into lesions or skin scarification at a site distant from the tumor |
| **C Parvum** (*Corynebacterium parvulum*) | Gram-positive aerobic of the tubercle bacillus | Subcutaneously or intravenously |
| **MER** (methanol extract residue) | Extracted residue of the tubercle bacillus | Intradermally or intralesionally |

## Using a Heaf gun to administer immunotherapy

**1** *Is immunotherapy with BCG part of your patient's treatment? You'll use a Heaf gun to administer the medication for several reasons: it gives you better control of needle penetration; it provides a more consistent immunization pattern; and it causes less pain and disfigurement than other immunotherapy methods. Do you know how to use the Heaf gun? If not, read this photostory.*

Obtain a tuberculin syringe, and attach a 22G needle to it. Then, draw up one vial of BCG vaccine that's been warmed at room temperature for 1 hour and reconstituted with 1 ml diluent. Gather the rest of the equipment you'll need: acetone, a 4" x 4" sterile gauze pad, sterile cotton balls, sterile gloves, 1" wide paper tape, and a sterilized Heaf gun (with needle cartridge).

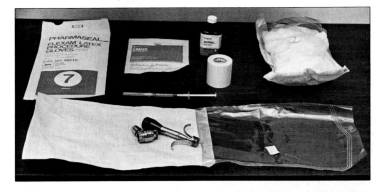

**4** Estimate the injection site's perimeters at about 3 cm sq. The standard vaccine application calls for four Heaf gun firings. Since two drops of vaccine are needed for each Heaf gun firing, use the drawn up syringe to put 8 drops of vaccine on the 3 cm sq site.

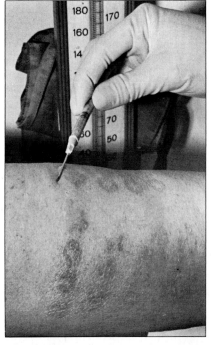

**2** Locate the injection site, as ordered by the doctor. Clean the area with acetone, and let it dry naturally. Position the patient so the site is as level as possible.

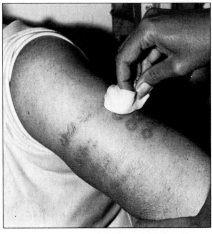

**5** Then, holding the patient's skin taut, press the Heaf gun on the site. You can fire it manually or set it to self-fire. Repeat the firing three more times, moving the gun across the site. If there's any BCG left in the syringe, spread it over the injected area, using the side of the needle.

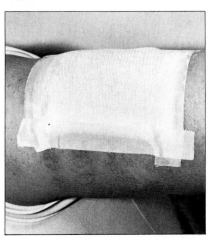

**3** Slip on sterile gloves. Then, assemble the Heaf gun by inserting the needle cartridge into the gun barrel and screwing on the plunger. Set the gun's penetration level at the NUMBER 2 setting (2 mm).

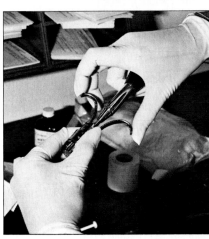

**6** Finally, let the site dry naturally. Cover it with the sterile gauze pad, and tape the pad securely. Do not remove the pad for 48 hours. Repeat the procedure as ordered. Don't let the site get wet for at least 6 weeks or until a crust forms over it.

☛ *Nursing tip:* You can cover BCG ulcerations with Vaseline or Vaseline gauze to prevent clothing from sticking to them.

# Subcutaneous administration

What's the first thing that pops into your mind when you hear the words subcutaneous injection? Do you think of a diabetic patient? Or perhaps of a patient suffering from an allergic reaction? The doctor could order a subcutaneous injection for either patient. But that's only part of it. Consider the following: Do you know there are eight different areas of the body suitable for giving a subcutaneous injection? Do you know which areas are the most common? Name several indications for giving medication subcutaneously. What are several of the reasons for *not* giving medication by this route? How can you help the diabetic maintain a systematic site rotation plan? What will happen if he doesn't?

As you can see, there's more to subcutaneous injections than you may have thought. Read the next several pages. In them, you'll not only discover the answers to these questions, but you'll also find important instructions and helpful tips for giving subcutaneous injections confidently.

### When to inject a drug subcutaneously

You'll give a medication subcutaneously when you want it to take effect slowly. Most subcutaneous medications are isotonic, nonirritating, nonviscous, and soluble. They're absorbed through both adipose and connective tissue.
*The doctor may order a subcutaneous injection if:*
• the medication works more effectively when it's absorbed through subcutaneous tissue.
• your patient can't or won't swallow.
• your patient can't take anything by mouth for any reason; for example, when he's vomiting or undergoing gastric suctioning.
• the medication's action would be destroyed by gastrointestinal secretions.
• the medication would irritate the gastrointestinal tract.

*But he won't order a subcutaneous injection if:*
• your patient is in shock.
• your patient has occlusive vascular disease, with poor perfusion.
• your patient's skin tissue is grossly adipose, edematous, burned, hardened, or swollen at all the common sites.
• your patient's skin tissue was damaged by previous injections.
• your patient's skin tissue is diseased.
• the drug isn't recommended for subcutaneous injection.

**Nurses' guide to subcutaneous injection sites**

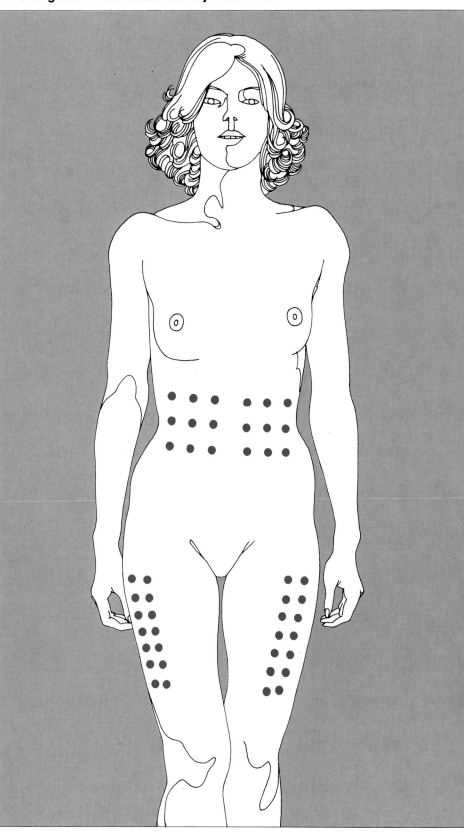

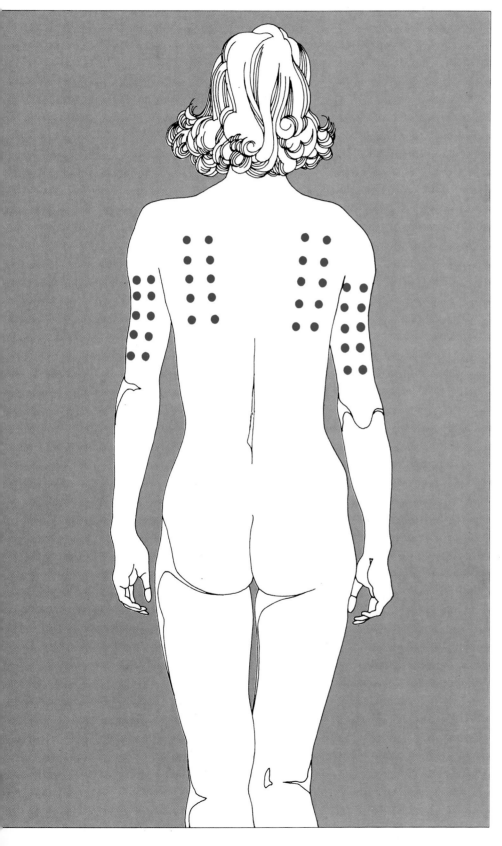

You can give a subcutaneous injection in any part of a patient's body where relatively few sensory nerve endings are present, and large blood vessels and bones aren't near the surface. The most common sites, shown in this illustration, are the outer aspects of the arms and thighs. Less common sites include the lower abdomen, above the iliac crest, and the upper back.

When you select an injection site, make sure it has a fat fold of at least 1" (2.5 cm) when you pinch the area between your thumb and forefinger. You'll find subcutaneous tissue abundant in well-nourished, well-hydrated patients and sparse in frail, cachexic, or dehydrated patients.

The absorption of medication given by any parenteral route is chiefly influenced by blood flow. Since the blood is minimal in subcutaneous tissue, the absorption rate is usually slow. But a few medications, such as heparin, defy this rule; they're absorbed through the subcutaneous tissue as rapidly as they are through intramuscular tissue.

Here are some other ways absorption is affected:
• The trauma of injection releases histamine into subcutaneous tissue, which decreases blood flow and *slows* absorption.
• Physical exertion increases blood flow in subcutaneous tissue, in turn speeding up the absorption rate.
• Normal connective tissue prevents medication from spreading indiscriminately and slows the absorption rate. But this slowing process is altered by the enzyme hyaluronidase, which works by breaking down hyaluronic acid, a basic substance of connective tissue. As the hyaluronidase level in the medication increases, so do the absorption and diffusion rates.
• A highly soluble medication is absorbed more quickly than a less soluble one.

# Subcutaneous administration

### Injecting medication subcutaneously

**1** *You're working in the ED, and Elsa Davenport comes in suffering an allergic reaction from a bee sting. You're instructed to administer 0.5 ml aqueous epinephrine 1:1,000 to her subcutaneously. Do you know how? If not, read on.*

Before you begin, gather the following equipment: the ordered medication; several alcohol swabs; a 1 cc syringe with a ⅝" needle attached; and an assortment of other needles, 25G to 27G in diameter and ½" to 1" in length.

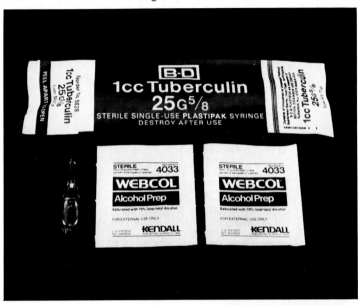

**2** Next, select the injection site, which in this case is the deltoid area of Mrs. Davenport's arm. To locate it exactly, position her arm by her side, inner aspect up. Then, measure 1 handbreadth down from the top of her shoulder and a third of the way around to the arm's outer aspect. As you work, explain the procedure to Mrs. Davenport.

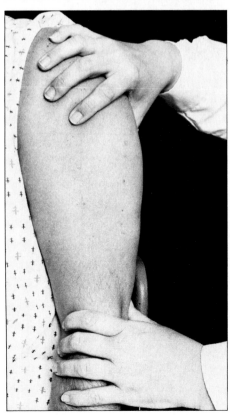

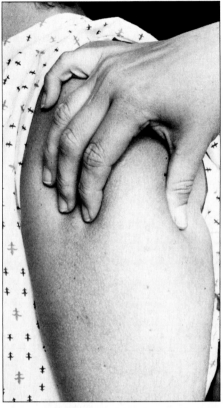

**3** Now you're ready to determine the exact needle size you need. To do this, use your thumb and forefinger to form a fold of skin at the site. Measure from the fold's base to its crest. If the fold measures more or less than ⅝" (1 cm), remove the ⅝" needle that's on the syringe, and replace it with one that's closer to the correct length. (You'll probably need a ½" needle for a child or a thin patient and a ⅞" or 1" needle for an overweight patient.)

By using a needle that's the correct length, you minimize the risk of missing the subcutaneous tissue. You also spare your patient unnecessary pain.

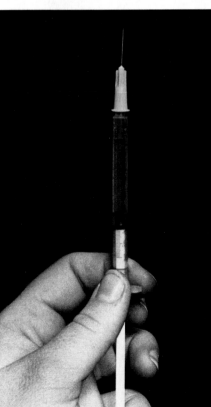

**4** Now, examine the medication. Make sure it's not outdated or contaminated. Then, break off the ampule's neck, as explained on page 62. Insert the needle into the ampule, and withdraw 0.5 ml of the medication. Then, pull back on the plunger to introduce a 0.2 to 0.3 cc air bubble into the syringe barrel, as shown here. Later, when you inject the medication, this bubble will help seal it in the subcutaneous tissue.

**5** Clean the injection site with an alcohol swab. To do this properly, begin at the center of the site and move outward in a circular motion. Allow the skin to dry completely before you proceed. If the skin's still wet when you inject the medication, you may introduce some of the alcohol into the subcutaneous tissue.

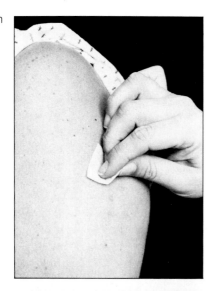

**6** Now, grasp the skin firmly, as the nurse is doing here. This elevates the subcutaneous tissue and prevents the needle from entering the wrong skin layer. Position the needle bevel up. If you're injecting with a ½" needle, hold it at a 90° angle to the skin. If you're using a ⅝" or longer needle, position it at a 45° angle, as shown here.

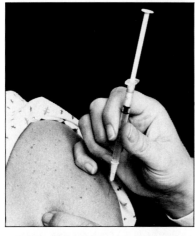

**7** Insert the needle in one quick motion. Once it's inserted, release your grasp on the patient's skin. If you don't, you'll inject into the compressed tissue, which'll irritate nerve fibers and cause discomfort for your patient.

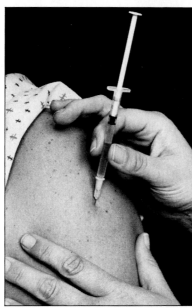

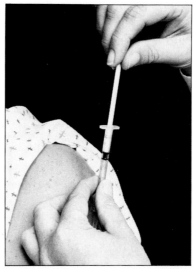

**8** Then, pull back slightly on the plunger to check needle placement. If you get a blood backflow, quickly withdraw the needle and place an alcohol swab over the site. Suppose the blood discolors the medication in the syringe. Discard everything and begin again. However, if the blood backflow is minimal, simply replace the needle with a sterile one, and insert it at a new site.

If there's no blood backflow, begin injecting the medication *slowly*. Never inject rapidly; doing so will put pressure on the tissue and cause pain.

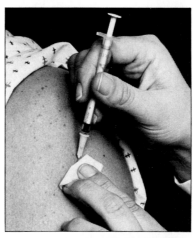

**9** When you've finished injecting, place an alcohol swab over the site. Then, withdraw the needle at the same angle you inserted it. As you do, use the swab to apply pressure to the site. Applying pressure will help seal punctured tissue and prevent medication seepage.

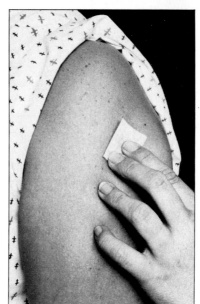

**10** Next, use a clean alcohol swab to massage the site. This will help distribute the medication and promote its absorption by dilating the blood vessels in the area and increasing blood flow.

Finally, document what you've done and your patient's response to it. Include the name of the prescribed drug; its dosage, route, site, time of administration; and your initials. Afterward, dispose of all equipment according to your hospital's policy.

# Subcutaneous administration

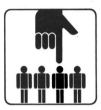

### What you should know about injecting heparin

To inject heparin, follow the usual procedure for any subcutaneous injection, except for these considerations:

- Use a ½" 25G or 26G needle.
- Select an injection site on the patient's abdomen just above the level of his anterior iliac spine, as shown in this illustration. Remember, you must rotate injection sites. Study this illustration to determine which sites to choose.
- Pinch a ½" (1.3 cm) fold of tissue between your thumb and forefinger, and insert the needle into the fold at a 90° angle. Using this technique will minimize heparin's irritating qualities. Applying ice to the site before injecting may help too. But don't apply it until you check your hospital's policy on this technique and have a doctor's order for it.
- Don't check for blood backflow. You could damage the tissue and cause a hematoma.
- Never massage the site after the injection. You could rupture the small blood vessels and cause a hematoma.

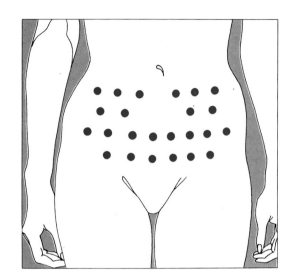

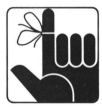

### Teaching the diabetic about injections

Teaching your diabetic patient how to rotate his injection sites systematically and mix his insulin (if necessary) are two of your most important responsibilities. Explain to him that if he fails to rotate the injection site, he could experience any of the following tissue complications:
- *Atrophy* (loss of subcutaneous fat). A small dimple or depression will form at the injection site, interfering with absorption. This can scar or desensitize the area.
- *Hypertrophy* (thickening of the subcutaneous tissue). The skin around the injection site will appear lumpy, hard, or spongy. This condition also interferes with absorption and can scar or desensitize the area. (Hypertrophy may also be caused by delivering cold insulin.)
- *Unabsorbed insulin deposits*. The patient will show signs of *hyperglycemia:* loss of appetite, lethargy, nausea, vomiting, high urine sugar, a positive urine acetone reading, frequent urination, and marked thirst.

But suppose he suddenly becomes more active or traumatizes the deposit. His subcutaneous circulation will increase, in turn increasing absorption and causing *hypoglycemia*.

To teach your patient how to rotate injection sites properly, have him choose one of the several site selection plans available. Clip a copy of his plan to his chart. Make sure the plan is followed, by documenting each site as it's used. If the patient or his family will be administering the insulin without your supervision, instruct them carefully. Then, give them a copy of the home care aid shown on the opposite page.

Suppose your diabetic patient must administer a combination of regular and NPH insulin. You must teach him how to draw them up in the same syringe without contaminating the vials. To do this, demonstrate the procedure by following these steps:
- Clean the top of both vials with alcohol.
- Draw air into the syringe in an amount equal to the prescribed dose of NPH insulin.
- Inject all the air into the NPH vial. Remove the syringe from the vial.
- Now, draw air into the syringe in an amount equal to the prescribed dose of regular insulin.
- Inject the air into the regular insulin vial. Then, invert the vial, and withdraw the prescribed dose of regular insulin.
- Before you remove the syringe, check for air bubbles in the syringe barrel. If any are present, lightly tap the syringe with your finger. (This will cause the bubbles to rise to the top.) Then, push up slightly on the plunger to force the air back into the vial. Make sure the syringe still contains the prescribed dose of insulin. If it doesn't, draw the amount you need. Then, withdraw the needle and syringe.
- Now, insert the needle into the NPH vial, and invert the vial. Withdraw the correct amount of NPH insulin. Be sure you don't push any regular insulin into the vial or you'll mix the regular insulin with the NPH insulin.

Here's an easy way to teach this mixing procedure to your patient: Take two empty vials, and fill one with water and the other with water tinted with red food coloring. Label the vial containing the tinted water REGULAR INSULIN. Label the other vial NPH INSULIN. Then, let the patient practice drawing up a combination of clear and colored water. You'll know at a glance if he's done the procedure correctly, because the water in the vial labeled NPH insulin will show no trace of red from the food coloring.

# Patient teaching

## Home care

### How to give yourself an insulin injection

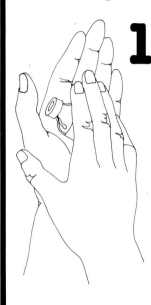

**1** Dear Patient:
This aid is meant to supplement, not replace, the instructions from your nurse. Use it as a written reminder of what the nurse has taught you. Before beginning the procedure, wash your hands thoroughly. Then, remove the insulin from the refrigerator. Warm and mix it by rolling the vial between your palms. Check the expiration date, and read the label to make sure the medication's the correct strength and type. Important: Never shake the vial.

Using an alcohol swab, cleanse the rubber stopper on top of the vial.

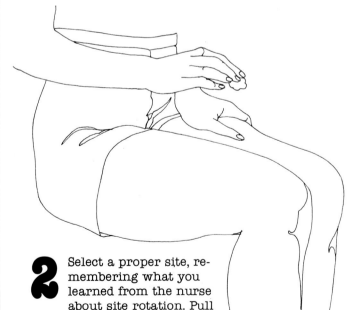

**2** Select a proper site, remembering what you learned from the nurse about site rotation. Pull the skin taut, and use an alcohol swab or a cotton ball soaked in alcohol to clean it in a circular motion.

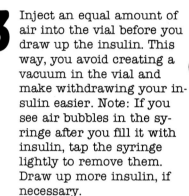

**3** Inject an equal amount of air into the vial before you draw up the insulin. This way, you avoid creating a vacuum in the vial and make withdrawing your insulin easier. Note: If you see air bubbles in the syringe after you fill it with insulin, tap the syringe lightly to remove them. Draw up more insulin, if necessary.

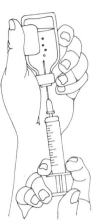

**4** Now, pinch the skin at the cleansed site between your thumb and forefinger. Quickly plunge the needle into the fat fold at a 90° angle, right up to its hub. As you hold the syringe with one hand, pull back on the plunger slightly with your other hand, to check for blood backflow. If blood appears in the syringe, discard everything and start again. If no blood appears, inject the insulin slowly.

**5** Place an alcohol swab over the site. Use the swab to press lightly on the site as you withdraw the needle. Snap the needle off the syringe. Dispose of the needle and syringe properly. The nurse will give you a guide that'll show you how to rotate your injection sites correctly. To help you remember, use a calendar to mark which site you plan to use for each day.

Important: If you travel, keep a bottle of insulin and a syringe with you at all times. The insulin doesn't need to be refrigerated if you keep it away from heat.

# Subcutaneous administration

## Helping visually impaired diabetics with special equipment

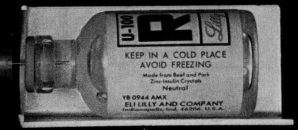

*Before beginning your teaching sessions with a diabetic patient, find out if he has impaired vision. Because many patients won't admit that they have trouble seeing, this can hinder your teaching efforts and jeopardize the therapy's effectiveness. Some of the devices available for the visually impaired or blind diabetic are shown here.*

### AFB needle guide

This metal guide is custom-cut to accommodate any size bottle of insulin. Here's how to use it: place the needle in the V-shaped notch. Then, lay the bottle in the trough so it faces the V-shaped notch. Push the bottle along the trough to insert the needle into the stopper.

Remember, once the notch is cut, this guide can only be used with one size bottle. Also, when this device is used, the needle can become easily contaminated.

### Dos-Aid Syringe Filling Device

This plastic device accommodates disposable U-100 syringes. The doctor will position the plunger stop at a point determined by the dose. Then he'll tighten the stop so it can't be moved, thereby governing the amount of insulin drawn up each time by the patient.

The Dos-Aid Syringe Filling Device has these disadvantages: it can only be used with one brand of syringe after the plunger stop has been secured; the needle can become easily contaminated; and the plunger stop may loosen and move with repeated use.

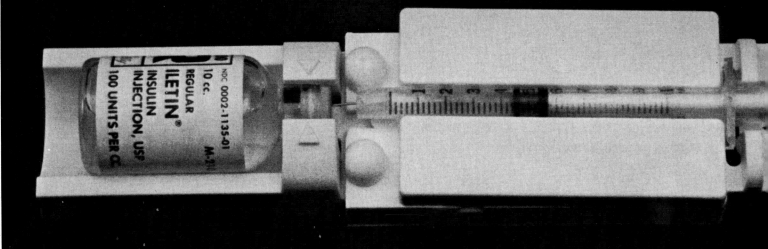

### Lilly needle guide

This small, funnel-shaped metal device fits over the top of insulin vials to help guide the needle into the rubber stopper. This needle guide works only with vials manufactured by the Eli Lilly Co.

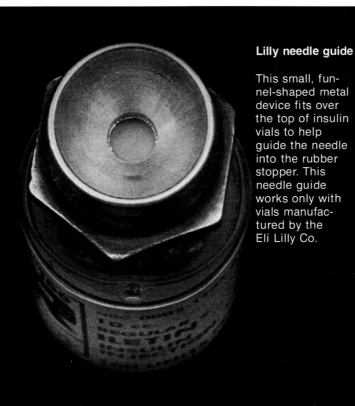

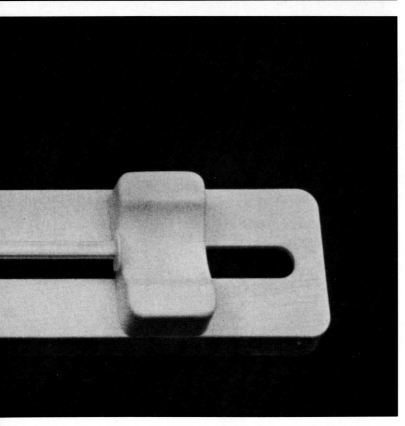

### Monoject scale magnifier

This small piece of plastic snaps into place on insulin syringes and enlarges the numbers on the barrel. However, arthritic patients may find this device difficult to attach.

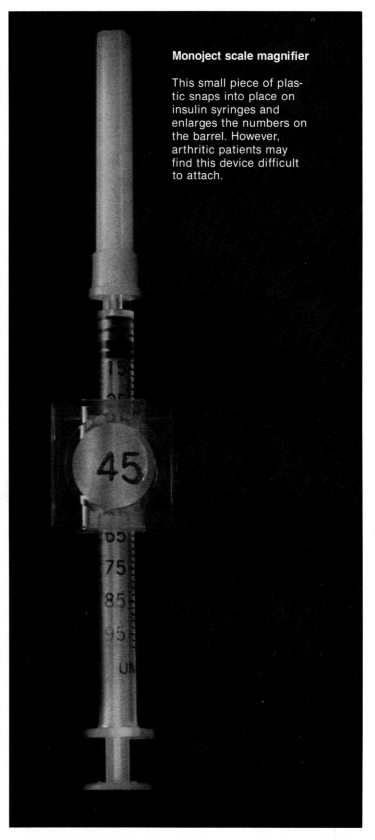

# Intramuscular administration

Let's imagine you're caring for a patient with tuberculosis. The doctor orders 1 g streptomycin sulfate to be given intramuscularly every 12 hours. Do you know how to do it? Aside from general skills, do you know the specific techniques for I.M. injection? For example, which site is best for your patient? When is the Z-track method indicated? What are the common problems connected with I.M. injections? These and other questions are answered on the following pages. Study them carefully.

## I.M. injections: Pros and cons

You'll give medication by the intramuscular route when you want to:
• administer aqueous suspensions, solutions in oil, or medications that don't come in oral form.
• administer parenteral medications in large doses (up to 5 ml).
• administer medication to a patient who's uncooperative, unconscious, or unable to swallow.
• avoid loss of drug effects from vomiting or gastric activity.
• achieve a rapid effect.
• ensure long-term absorption by forming a medication deposit.
   The advantages of using the intramuscular route over other parenteral routes are that muscles contain more blood vessels and have fewer sensory nerve endings. But the disadvantages include these risks:
• You may damage blood vessels, causing bleeding or improper routing of medication.
• You may damage nerves, causing unnecessary pain or paralysis.
• You may damage bone.

## Nurses' guide to intramuscular injection sites

When you're giving an intramuscular injection, you have five basic sites to choose from. The absorption rate for each site is about the same. Intramuscular absorption is similar to, but more rapid than, subcutaneous absorption because of increased blood flow to the muscles. For example, aqueous medications are absorbed from a muscle site within 10 to 30 minutes, while it takes over 30 minutes from a subcutaneous site.
   Keep in mind, however, not all intramuscular medications take effect at the same speed. Study the following illustrations to determine which site is best for your patient.

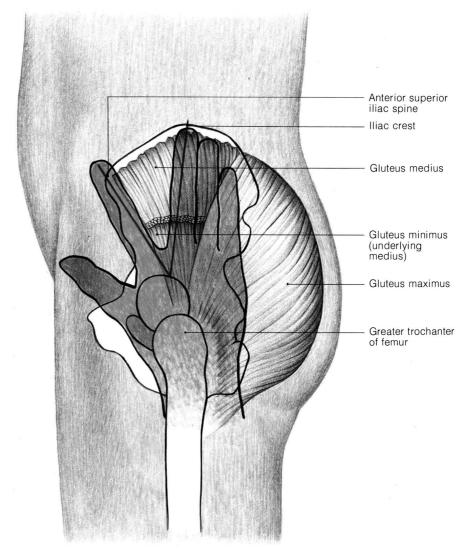

Anterior superior iliac spine
Iliac crest
Gluteus medius
Gluteus minimus (underlying medius)
Gluteus maximus
Greater trochanter of femur

**Ventrogluteal**

Used for all patients. Desirable because the site is not only relatively free of large nerves and fat tissue, but remote from rectum (which minimizes the risk of contamination).

Position patient on his back or side.

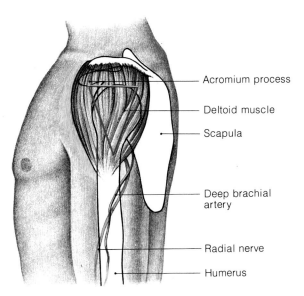

- Acromium process
- Deltoid muscle
- Scapula
- Deep brachial artery
- Radial nerve
- Humerus

### Deltoid

Seldom used because the muscle is small and can accommodate only small doses. It's also dangerously near the radial nerve.

Seat patient upright or have him lie flat, with his arms apart.

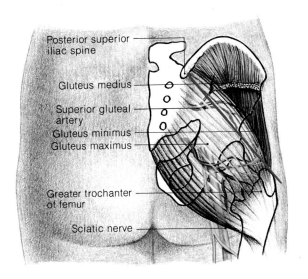

- Posterior superior iliac spine
- Gluteus medius
- Superior gluteal artery
- Gluteus minimus
- Gluteus maximus
- Greater trochanter of femur
- Sciatic nerve

### Dorsogluteal

Commonly used for adults, but not for infants and children under age 3 because their dorsogluteal muscles aren't well developed.

Position patient flat on his stomach, with his toes pointed inward, and his arms apart and flexed toward his head.

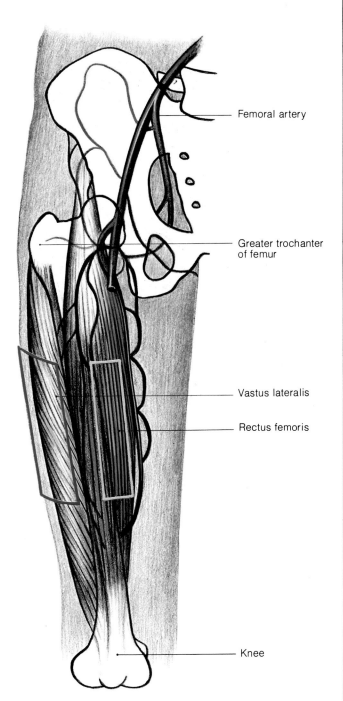

- Femoral artery
- Greater trochanter of femur
- Vastus lateralis
- Rectus femoris
- Knee

### Vastus lateralis and rectus femoris

The vastus lateralis is used for all patients, especially children. It's well developed and has few major blood vessels and nerves. The rectus femoris is most often used for self-injection because of its accessibility.

Position patient in bed either sitting up or lying flat.

# Intramuscular administration

### Injecting medication intramuscularly

**1** *Bertha Nelan, a 39-year-old schoolteacher, has pneumonia. As part of her treatment, the doctor has ordered 500 mg ampicillin sodium (Amcill-S) I.M. every 6 hours. It's time to give her an injection. Do you know how?*

First, wash your hands. Remember to maintain sterile technique throughout the procedure. Then, gather your equipment: medication, the diluent, a 3 cc syringe, a 22G 1½" needle, and several alcohol swabs.

Examine the medication vial. Make sure it's not outdated or contaminated. Then, explain to the patient what you're going to do.

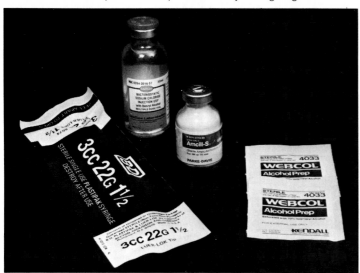

**2** Now you're ready to prepare the medication. Reconstitute it, following the procedure on page 62. Then, swab the stopper on the medication vial with alcohol. Attach the needle to the syringe, and insert it into the stopper. Draw up 500 mg ampicillin. Then, draw up 0.2 to 0.3 cc air. This air bubble will help clear the medication from the needle when you inject. It'll also prevent medication seepage from the site afterward.

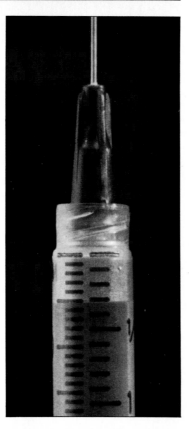

**3** You decide to use the vastus lateralis site for the injection. To expose the site, position Mrs. Nelan on her back.

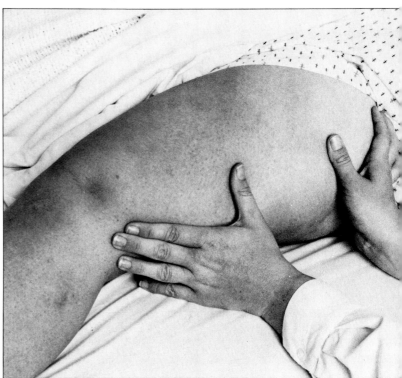

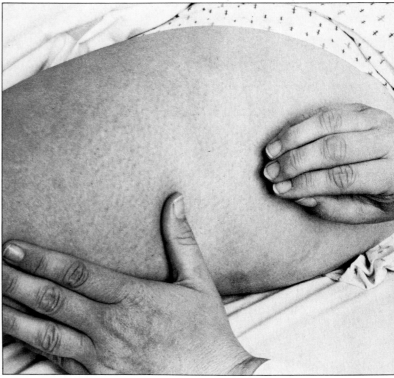

**4** Gently tap the site, as shown here. This will stimulate the nerve endings and minimize initial pain when the needle's inserted.

**5** Clean a 2" (5 cm) diameter area around the injection site, moving from the center outward in a circular motion. This will reduce the chance of introducing pathogens into the tissue when you penetrate the skin with the needle. Place the swab between two of your fingers for later use. Let the alcohol dry before you inject, so you don't force any of it into the subcutaneous tissue.

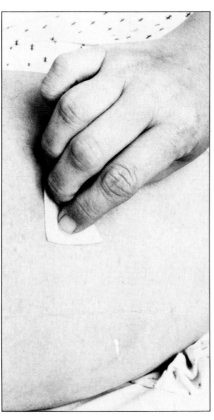

**7** Use your other hand to hold the syringe. Make sure you keep it horizontal until you're ready to inject. Doing so will prevent gravity from altering the plunger's position.

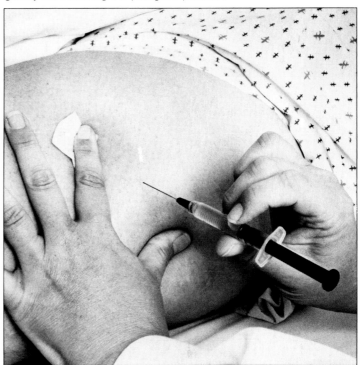

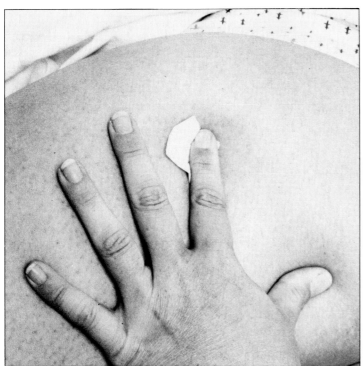

**6** With one hand, stretch the skin around the injection site so it's taut. Beside making needle insertion easier, this displaces subcutaneous tissue, which helps disperse the medication.

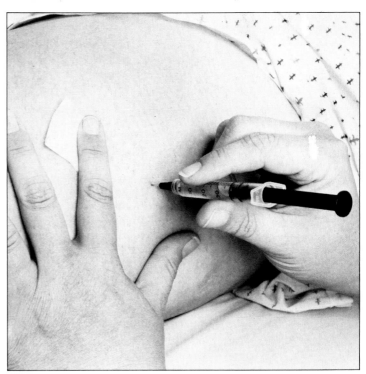

**8** Insert the needle at a 90° angle, with a quick, dart-like thrust. (Expect to feel some resistance.) This quick thrust facilitates needle entry and minimizes pain.

# Intramuscular administration

**9** Gently pull back on the plunger to confirm correct needle placement. If blood appears in the syringe, you may have punctured a vein. Withdraw the needle, replace it with a new one, and try again. If no blood appears, continue to the next step.

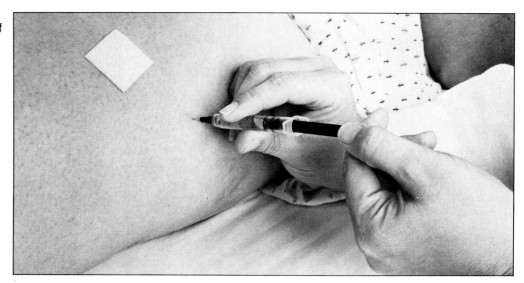

**10** Hold the needle steady to avoid traumatizing the tissue. Then, inject the medication at a slow, even rate. If you force it, you'll hurt your patient unnecessarily and cause improper drug distribution.

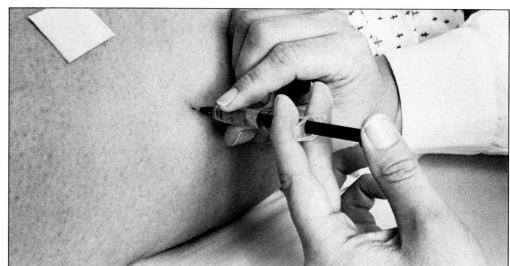

**11** When you've finished injecting, withdraw the needle rapidly. Use an alcohol swab to apply pressure to the site. As you continue to apply pressure, massage the site with a circular motion. This will distribute the medication over a greater area. *Note:* Don't massage the site when you want slow absorption or when you're delivering an extremely irritating medication, like cefazolin sodium (Ancef*). Instead, just apply pressure.

Watch for adverse effects immediately following the injection and up to 30 minutes afterward. Document the following: medication given, route, site, amount, time, patient's reaction, and your initials. Finally, discard the equipment according to your hospital's policies. Be sure to wash your hands afterward.

*Available in the United States and in Canada.

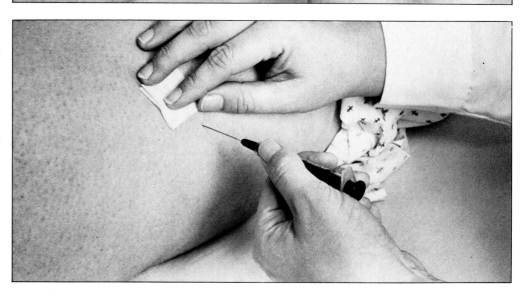

## Using the Z-track method for injection

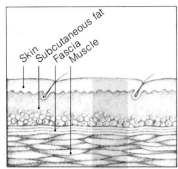

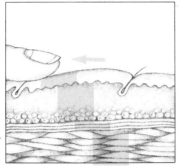

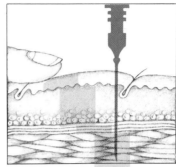

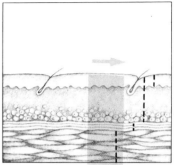

**1** *If you're administering iron dextran complex (Imferon\*), you must vary the standard injection procedure by performing what's known as the Z-track method.* It involves pulling the skin in such a way that the needle track is sealed off after the injection. Doing this minimizes subcutaneous irritation and discoloration.

You'll inject the drug into the patient's buttock. To find out how, read on.

**2** After drawing up 0.3 to 0.5 cc of air into the syringe, replace the needle with a sterile one that's 3" (7.6 cm) long.

Pull the skin laterally away from the intended injection site. This will ensure proper entry of muscle tissue.

**3** After cleansing the site, insert the needle, and inject the medication slowly.

When you've completed the injection, wait for 10 seconds before you withdraw the needle. This way you'll prevent medication seepage from the site.

**4** Withdraw the needle and syringe. Now, allow the retracted skin to resume its normal position. This will effectively seal off the needle track.

Never massage the site or allow the patient to wear tight-fitting clothes. Otherwise, the medication could be forced into the subcutaneous tissue and cause irritation.

To increase the absorption rate, encourage physical activity; for example, walking. For subsequent injections, alternate buttocks.

## Problems caused by improper technique

COMPLICATIONS

Study this chart to learn how you can minimize your patient's pain from intramuscular injections.

| Improper technique | Result | Possible complications |
|---|---|---|
| Using incorrect length needle | Injecting into wrong skin layer | • Nonspecific injection pain<br>• Sterile abscess<br>• Tissue degeneration<br>• Granuloma<br>• Hypertrophy |
| Forgetting to replace needle between drawing up medication and injecting | Medication adhering to outside of needle | • Nonspecific injection pain<br>• Tissue discoloration with iron dextran complex (Imferon\*) |
| Not locating proper landmarks before injecting | Pushing needle against a nerve or injecting into a blood vessel | • Shooting pain down limb<br>• Paralysis<br>• Bleeding |
| Forgetting to check for blood backflow | Injecting into a vein | • Speed shock (increased heart rate, shortness of breath, decreased blood pressure, loss of consciousness) |
| Neglecting to draw 0.2 to 0.3 cc air into syringe before injecting | Medication leaking from injection site | • Skin irritation<br>• Formation of a lump under the skin |

\*Available in the United States and in Canada.

# Intravenous administration

If you've ever performed I.V. therapy, you know it's more involved than just putting a needle in your patient's arm. The following pages will answer your questions about:
• performing venipuncture
• using the bolus method
• using the drip method
• I.V. therapy complications
• drugs that require special procedures
• plus much, much more.

Keep in mind, however, that I.V. therapy is so complex we can only cover the basics here. For details on all the topics that follow, refer to the NURSING PHOTOBOOK *Managing I.V. Therapy.*

## When to give medications intravenously

*You'll administer medications intravenously when you want to:*
• immediately treat life-threatening conditions, such as acute epiglottitis or shock.
• quickly achieve and maintain the proper drug level in the patient's bloodstream.
• deliver medications that can't be given by any other route, such as dopamine hydrochloride (Intropin*).
• deliver large doses of medication, such as carbenicillin disodium (Geopen).
• treat the patient who can't receive medications by any other route; for example, a patient who has gastric ulcers or one who's unconscious.
• avoid damaging subcutaneous or intramuscular layers with potentially harmful drugs, such as levarterenol (Levophed*).
• delay drug deactivation by the liver.

*Don't administer medication intravenously if:*
• the medication comes in an oral form and the patient can swallow it.
• the patient has a blood coagulation disorder (unless, of course, the medication's needed to treat the condition).

*Available in the United States and in Canada.

**Dorsum of the hand**

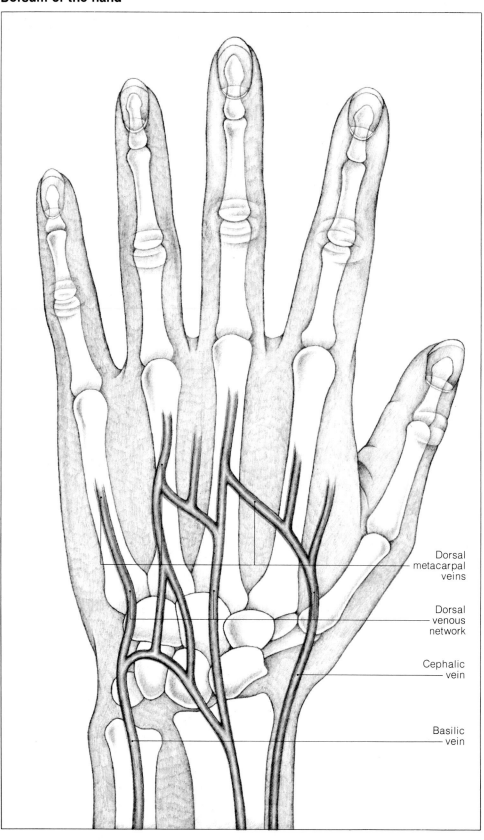

Dorsal metacarpal veins

Dorsal venous network

Cephalic vein

Basilic vein

## Choosing the correct venipuncture site

You've been instructed to give your patient medication intravenously, so you'll have to perform venipuncture. Do you know which site is best for your patient?

In most cases, the best sites for venipuncture on a patient are (in order of preference) his lower arm and hand, his upper arm, and his antecubital fossa. Avoid performing venipuncture in the patient's legs, because he'll run a greater risk of developing thrombophlebitis and an embolism. Whenever possible, use the distal end of the vein. But first, ask yourself these questions:

• **How long will I.V. therapy last?** For short-term therapy, use the patient's left arm or hand if he's right-handed, his right arm or hand if he's left-handed. For long-term therapy, alternate the patient's arms and avoid sites over joints.

 *Nursing tip:* If your patient will be receiving long-term I.V. therapy, get maximum use from his arm veins by starting the therapy in a hand vein, then switching to sites farther up his arm, as necessary.

• **What kind of I.V. solution's been ordered?** For infusions that are highly acidic, alkaline, or hypertonic, use a large vein to adequately dilute the infusion. A small peripheral vein may become irritated. Rapid infusions also require larger veins.

• **What size needle or cannula are you using?** If the solution's highly viscous, you'll need a large-bore needle or cannula.

Then, choose a vein that's big enough to accommodate it.

• **Is the vein full, soft, and unobstructed?** Palpate the patient's veins to find one that's not crooked, hardened, scarred, or inflamed. If you must perform venipuncture in one of the patient's legs, avoid using a varicose vein. However, if you *must* use one, elevate the patient's leg during the infusion.

What if the patient's veins are neither visible nor palpable? You may find a fiberoptic illuminator helpful. To use it, turn off the room lights, and put the illuminator probe under the patient's palm. His hand will appear red and the veins black.

• **Does your patient have any specific problems or injuries that require special consideration?** Avoid veins in irritated, infected, or injured areas. The added stress of venipuncture may cause complications. If the patient's had a radical mastectomy, don't start an I.V. in the arm on that side of her body.

• **How old is the patient?** If your patient's an adolescent or an adult, his hand or lower arm will probably provide the best site. But if you're giving I.V. therapy to an infant, insert the needle in a scalp vein, where it can be protected. Then, cover the site with an inverted paper cup that's been slotted on one side to accommodate the tube. Tape the cup to the infant's head with nonallergenic tape.

## I.V. administration methods: How they differ

**Direct** (I.V. bolus)
To deliver drugs rapidly

**Advantages**
• Drug becomes effective immediately, because it's injected directly into patient's bloodstream.
• Absorption process more predictable than with other methods.

**Disadvantages**
• May cause speed shock
• More likely to irritate vein
• Increases risk of complications, including extravasation, systemic infection, air embolism

---

**Continuous drip**
(primary line infusion)
To maintain delivery at a therapeutic level

**Advantages**
• Less irritating than bolus injection
• Requires less mixing and hanging than with intermittent method
• Easy to discontinue

**Disadvantages**
• Can be dangerous if I.V. flow rate isn't carefully monitored
• Many drugs don't remain stable for the length of time this method requires.
• Increases risk of complications, including extravasation, systemic infection, air embolism
• Mixing medications may cause incompatibility.

---

**Intermittent** (additive set infusion)
To administer drugs mixed with diluent. May be infused intermittently over a period of time or as a one-time dose.

**Advantages**
• Administration time longer than bolus injection and shorter than continuous drip therapy.
• Less likely to cause speed shock than bolus injection
• Less irritating to veins than bolus injection

**Disadvantages**
• Expensive
• Increased chance of contamination with frequent port use
• Mixing medications may cause incompatibility.
• Increases risk of complications, including extravasation, systemic infection, air embolism

### Antecubital fossa

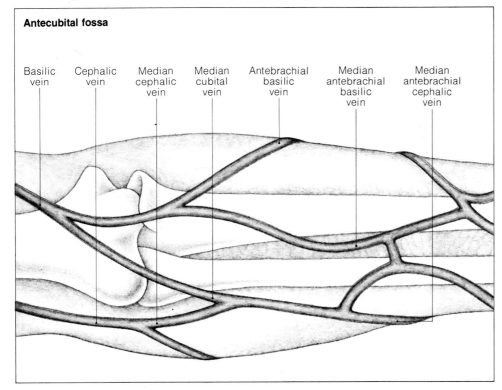

Basilic vein
Cephalic vein
Median cephalic vein
Median cubital vein
Antebrachial basilic vein
Median antebrachial basilic vein
Median antebrachial cephalic vein

# Intravenous administration

### Performing venipuncture

**1** *Preparing to give intravenous medication to your patient? Whether you use the bolus or the drip method, you'll have to perform venipuncture. Here's how:*

Begin by washing your hands and gathering the necessary equipment: an alcohol swab, a tourniquet, Betadine skin prep, antimicrobial ointment, a 2" x 2" sterile gauze pad, tape, and a needle or cannula. Since you'll probably be using an intermittent infusion set with a winged-tip needle, we've chosen to feature it in this photostory.

Explain the procedure to the patient. Then, get ready to insert the needle into his vein, using the easy, indirect method.

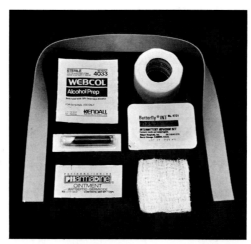

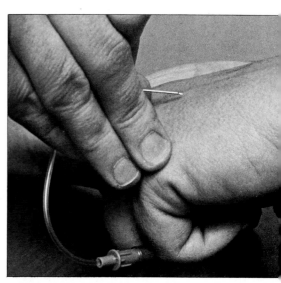

**2** First, select a vein. Apply a tourniquet to make it rise. Swab the site with Betadine, starting at the center and working outward in a circular motion. Clean an area about 2" (5 cm) in diameter.

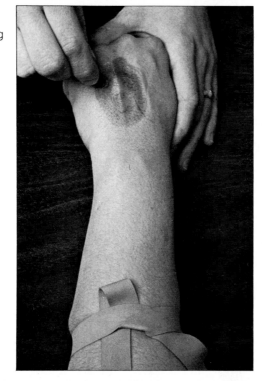

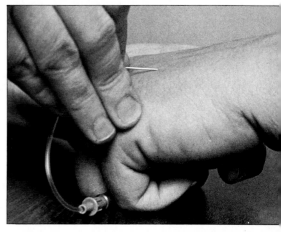

**3** Stabilize the dilated vein by anchoring it with your thumb and stretching the skin downward, as shown here. Is the vein you've selected in the patient's hand? You may find it helps to flex his wrist. Or ask the patient to help stabilize his vein by first making a fist with his free hand, then clasping it with the hand you're about to puncture.

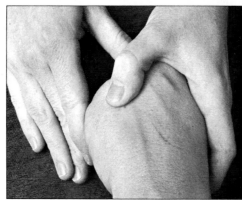

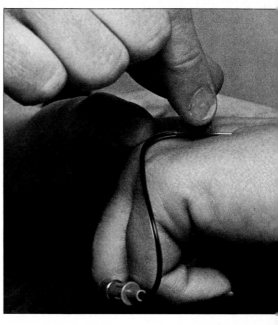

**4** When you've completed these steps, remove the needle guard. Point the needle in the direction of the blood flow, and hold it at a 45° angle above the skin, with the bevel facing up. Now, you're ready to insert the needle into the vein, using what's commonly called the indirect method of venipuncture.

**5** Here's how to do it: Pinch the wings together tightly. Keeping your hand steady, pierce the patient's skin at a point slightly to one side of the vein, and about ½" (1.3 cm) below the spot where you plan to puncture the vein wall.
 *Nursing tip:* To reduce the patient's discomfort during this step, ask him to inhale as you pierce his skin.

**6** Now, decrease the angle until the needle's almost level with the skin surface; then direct it toward the selected vein. You'll feel very little resistance as the needle goes through subcutaneous tissue. You'll feel considerably more resistance when you reach the vein.

Proceeding carefully, puncture the vein with the needle. Watch for blood backflow to confirm correct placement. Continue to advance the needle until it's well within the vein. By exerting a gentle, lifting pressure during this step, you can keep the needle from piercing the vein's opposite wall.
 *Nursing tip:* You can also puncture the vein with the one-step, or direct, method. To do so, dilate the vein as before. Insert the needle into the vein with one quick motion. Keep in mind, however, that this method requires more skill than the indirect method. Don't try it unless you've had some practice.

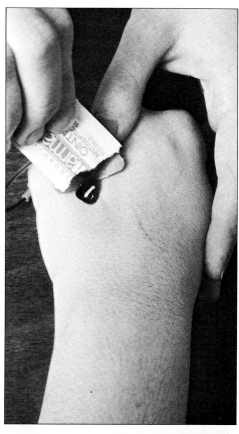

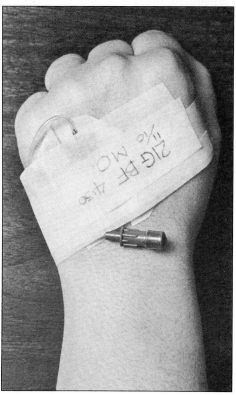

**7** Apply antimicrobial ointment to the venipuncture site. Then tape down a 2" x 2" sterile gauze pad. Also, secure the needle with tape. To do this, place one strip of tape over each wing, keeping the tape parallel to the needle. Then, place another strip of tape (perpendicular to the first two) directly on top of the wings, or just below them, on top of the tubing. Use whichever way lends more stability.
 *Nursing tip:* If you prefer, tape the needle down *before* you apply antimicrobial ointment and the 2" x 2" sterile gauze pad. This way, you can examine the site just by removing the bandage. For other common taping methods, see the NURSING PHOTOBOOK *Managing I.V. Therapy.*

**8** Next, loop the tubing, and secure the injection port with more tape. Don't make the loop so small that you kink it and restrict the fluid flow. Finally, label the site with the necessary information. Take a strip of tape and write the following information on it: date and time of insertion, type and gauge of needle, and your initials. Place it over the dressing. Don't apply the tape and then label it, or you'll irritate the site.

When you've completed the dressing label, make sure the container and tubing are labeled properly. Document the entire procedure in your notes.

# Intravenous administration

## Using the direct bolus method

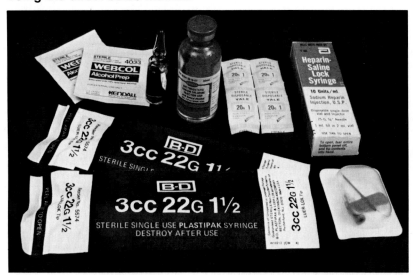

**1** *Mrs. Keppler has congestive heart failure. As part of her treatment, the doctor has ordered a 0.5 mg dose of digoxin (Lanoxin\*) to be delivered stat by I.V. bolus (commonly called I.V. push). How is it done? Read on.*

First, assemble the necessary equipment. You'll need the ordered medication, several syringes, several 1" needles, alcohol swabs, and an intermittent infusion set (heparin lock). You'll also need heparin or normal saline solution (depending on your hospital's policy) to flush the set after the injection.

Check the medication label against the Kardex to make sure it's correct. Also make sure the medication's not outdated or contaminated. If everything's in order, you're ready to draw the medication and the flushing solutions into syringes.

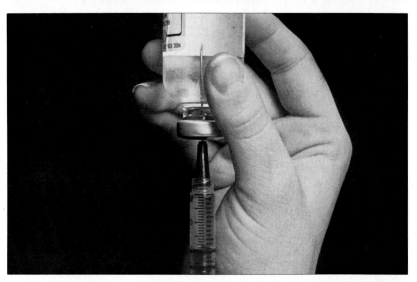

**2** Fill one syringe with heparin in the amount directed by hospital policy. This amount can range anywhere between 10 and 100 units. Fill another syringe with 2 ml saline solution, if hospital policy requires it, and a third syringe with the medication. Remember, use a filter needle to draw up the medication. Then, replace the filter needle with a regular needle.

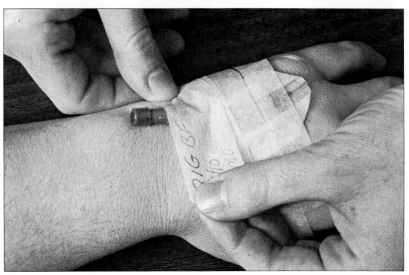

**3** If there's no intermittent infusion set already inserted in Mrs. Keppler's arm, prepare for venipuncture. First, explain the procedure to her. Then, apply a tourniquet. Make sure you select a large vein, to provide greater dilution and minimize irritation. Insert the intermittent infusion set into Mrs. Keppler's vein, following the procedure on pages 86 and 87.

Why use an intermittent infusion set instead of injecting directly into Mrs. Keppler's vein with the medication syringe? For three reasons: First, you'll save Mrs. Keppler the pain of repeated venipuncture, since she'll be receiving more than one medication by injection. Second, you'll reduce the risk of traumatizing the vein with a large needle. And third, you'll have less difficulty stabilizing the infusion set needle. Use tape to secure the set's injection port as far from the venipuncture site as possible. This further reduces the risk of moving the needle during the injection. Dress and label the site as usual.

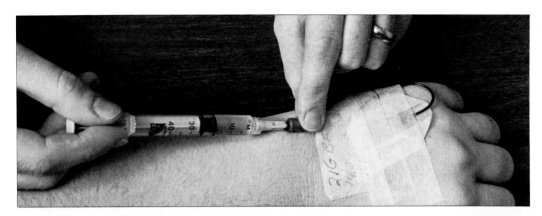

**4** Swab the injection port with alcohol. Insert the needle of the medication syringe into the port. Steady the hand that's holding the syringe by resting it on Mrs. Keppler's arm or on some nearby support.

Then, check the syringe for blood backflow. If none's present, withdraw the intermittent infusion set needle and reinsert it. If you do get a blood backflow, proceed to the next step.

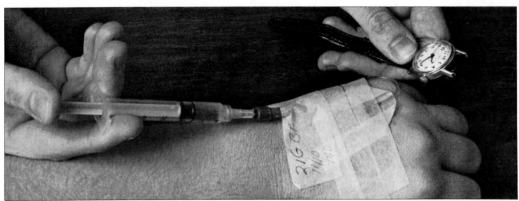

**5** Begin injecting the medication at the prescribed rate. To determine how much to infuse per minute, divide the prescribed dosage by the prescribed administration time. This will give you the correct amount.

*Important:* If you're delivering a toxic medication like fluorouracil (5-FU*), pull back on the plunger a few times during the injection to fill the syringe with blood. This serves two purposes: the blood backflow confirms correct needle placement and the blood itself helps dilute the medication.

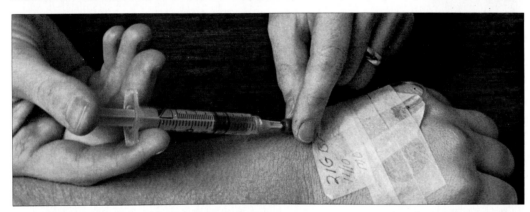

**6** Now, depending on your hospital's policy, do one or both of the following steps: Withdraw the medication syringe, and insert the needle of the saline-filled syringe in its place. Flush out any medication that remains in the intermittent infusion set.

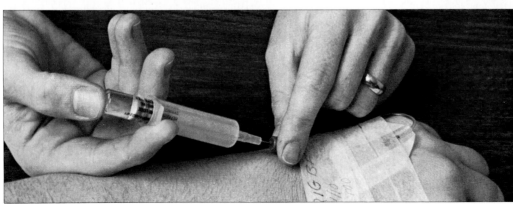

**7** Next, swab the port with alcohol. Insert the heparin-filled syringe, and inject the heparin solution. This will keep the I.V. tubing patent and will prepare the intermittent infusion set for reuse. (Replace the set with a new one every 2 days or as frequently as your hospital policy directs.)

Want to learn more about the I.V. bolus method for administering medications? Then read pages 81 to 87 in the NURSING PHOTOBOOK *Managing I.V. Therapy.*

*Available in the United States and in Canada.

# Intravenous administration

## Using the drip method

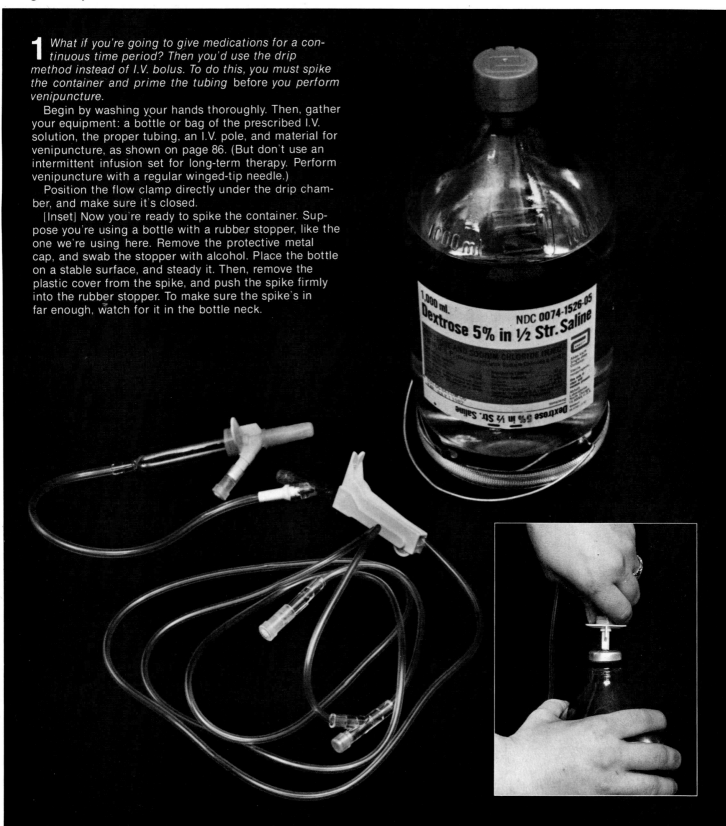

**1** *What if you're going to give medications for a continuous time period? Then you'd use the drip method instead of I.V. bolus. To do this, you must spike the container and prime the tubing before you perform venipuncture.*

Begin by washing your hands thoroughly. Then, gather your equipment: a bottle or bag of the prescribed I.V. solution, the proper tubing, an I.V. pole, and material for venipuncture, as shown on page 86. (But don't use an intermittent infusion set for long-term therapy. Perform venipuncture with a regular winged-tip needle.)

Position the flow clamp directly under the drip chamber, and make sure it's closed.

[Inset] Now you're ready to spike the container. Suppose you're using a bottle with a rubber stopper, like the one we're using here. Remove the protective metal cap, and swab the stopper with alcohol. Place the bottle on a stable surface, and steady it. Then, remove the plastic cover from the spike, and push the spike firmly into the rubber stopper. To make sure the spike's in far enough, watch for it in the bottle neck.

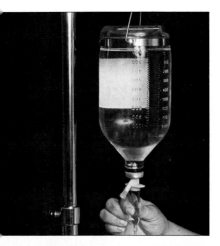

**2** Hang the container on an I.V. pole. Gently squeeze the drip chamber until it's half full. If you prime the tubing without doing this first, air bubbles may form in the drip chamber and travel down the tubing.

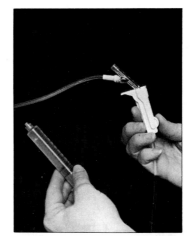

**5** What if you want to add medication to the solution after you've hung it on the I.V. pole? First, remove the needle from the medication syringe. Then, stop the flow to the patient by closing the clamp. Don't neglect this important step. Doing so could create a medication bolus, which may endanger your patient's life.

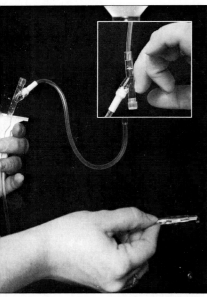

**3** Here's how to prime the tubing. First, hold the lower end of the tubing over a sink or wastebasket. Remove the protective cap. (Take care not to contaminate the cap, because you'll use it again.)

Now unclamp the tubing. Let the fluid run, as shown in this photo, until it fills the tubing and all air bubbles have been expelled. If you see small bubbles near the top of the tubing or in the drip chamber, lightly tap the area until the bubbles rise into the container.

[Inset] If the tubing has a backcheck valve, invert the valve as you prime. Gently tap the valve with your finger to remove air bubbles.

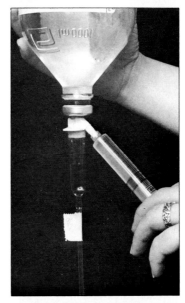

**6** Next, detach the air vent from the I.V. spike. But take care not to touch the ends and contaminate it. Then, as this photo shows, insert the syringe into the air vent port, and inject the medication.

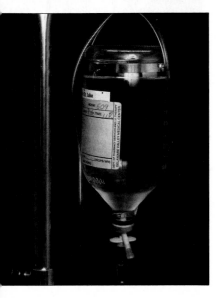

**4** Clamp the tubing, and replace the protective cap. Loop the tubing over the I.V. pole, so it's out of the way while you perform venipuncture, following the method described on pages 86 and 87. Label the container and tubing with the date and time of insertion.

When venipuncture's completed, uncap the I.V. tubing and attach it to the needle adapter. Open the flow clamp to begin the infusion into your patient. Time the flow rate with your wristwatch, and adjust the rate, if necessary.

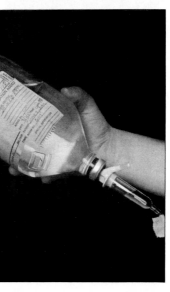

**7** Now, replace the air vent, and gently rotate the container to mix the solution. Finally, open the flow clamp, and adjust the flow rate. Label the bottle with the added medication, time and date of addition, and your initials. Document the entire procedure.

# Intravenous administration

## The drip method: Using a vented bottle or a bag

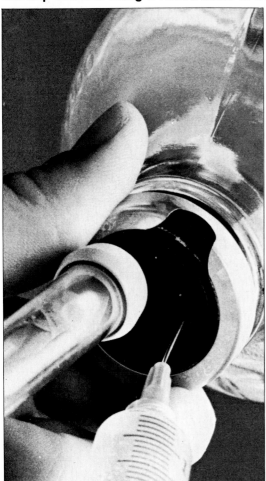

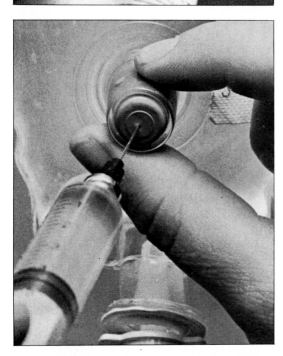

We've just shown you how to spike, prime, and add medication to a nonvented bottle. But what if you're using a vented bottle or bag? Each requires special consideration on your part. We'll explain the basics here. But for complete details you should refer to the NURSING PHOTOBOOK *Managing I.V. Therapy.*

**Vented bottle**
If you're using a bottle with an in-dwelling vent, like the one pictured to the left, follow these special instructions:
• Listen for a hiss of inrushing air when you remove the bottle's diaphragm. This confirms that the bottle's vacuum was intact. If you don't hear a hiss, the bottle is contaminated. Discard and replace it.
• To add medication to the bottle, clean the diaphragm with alcohol. Inject the medication through the printed triangle.
• Spike the bottle with *nonvented* tubing. To do this, insert the spike into the larger of the two holes in the bottle's stopper—the one *without* an air vent.
• Suppose you want to add medication to a bottle that's already hanging. First, make sure there's enough I.V. fluid to dilute the medication correctly. Then, follow the same procedure that's discussed above.

**Bag**
If you're using a bag, like the one shown on the left, follow these special instructions:
• Hang the bag *before* spiking. Then, when you pull off the cap, you're less likely to release the air needed to read the fluid level accurately.
*Note:* This rule doesn't apply to bags with an easy-grip port. Spike them as you would a bottle.
• Pull off the bag's cap in a smooth motion to the right. Pulling it to the left may rip it in two.
• Spike the bag with *nonvented* tubing, using a quick, smooth motion. If you hesitate, you may allow some of the I.V. solution to escape.
• Don't add medication to the bag once it's hanging *unless* there's enough solution in it for correct dilution. If there is enough solution, inject the medication through the injection port, observing the same aseptic techniques as you would for a bottle.

**When a child needs I.V. therapy**

A child receiving I.V. therapy needs your special care. Why? The procedure will probably be new and frightening for him. In addition, his anatomy and physiology differ significantly from an adult's.

Consider his size and metabolism rate, for example. A child's size increases the risk of both fluid and medication overdoses, and decreases his ability to overcome them if they occur. Second, a child's metabolism rate is about three times faster than an adult's. Because this rate determines the body's water requirements, a child needs more water per kg body weight than an adult and can easily become dehydrated.

The doctor considers these factors (along with the child's weight, size, and condition) when he calculates the amount to be administered intravenously. You can help him by taking baseline readings, keeping accurate intake and output records, and watching for complications. Keep in mind that changes can occur rapidly in children. Make sure your records are up to date.

You'll administer pediatric I.V. medication by the direct bolus method or with a volume-control set. A volume-control set is an I.V. line featuring a fluid chamber. This fluid chamber allows you to accurately deliver medications that you've diluted in precise amounts of fluid. When you use a volume-control set, make every effort to deliver all the medication in the fluid chamber. To ensure correct flow rate, use an infusion pump.

How can you help your young patient cope with his fears? Explain the procedure in words he can understand. Answer his questions honestly. Give him all the attention and support you can. (For more details on how to help the child who's about to undergo I.V. therapy, see the NURSING PHOTOBOOK *Managing I.V. Therapy.* Look for the specially designed children's coloring booklet on page 152. This patient teaching aid will help you explain what I.V. therapy's all about.)

### Understanding piggyback and secondary sets

The doctor will instruct you to connect a piggyback set or a secondary set to a primary I.V. line when he wants to:
- maintain peak drug levels in the patient's bloodstream.
- administer different drugs at different times.
- avoid vein irritation from I .V. bolus.

He won't order these methods if the drug you're administering must be given slowly or well diluted.

How does he choose between a piggyback set and a secondary set? Actually, the two terms are used interchangeably when nurses talk about any set that's added to a primary I.V. line. But, piggyback and secondary sets differ in purpose and design.

For example, you'll use a piggyback set solely for intermittent drug administration. This set features a small I.V. bottle (under 500 ml),

short tubing, and usually a macrodrip system. The piggyback bottle is hung above the primary I.V. container. (The manufacturer provided an extension hook so you can lower the primary container.) The tubing connects to the upper Y-port of a primary I.V. line. This port's usually called the piggyback port.

A secondary set is used to administer drugs intermittently or simultaneously with the primary I.V. solution. This set features an I.V. bottle (any size), long tubing, and either a microdrip or a macrodrip system. The secondary bottle should be hung at the same height as the primary container. The tubing connects to the primary line's lower Y-port, also called the secondary port.

For more information on piggyback and secondary sets, see the NURSING PHOTOBOOK *Managing I.V. Therapy.*

### Using a piggyback I.V. set

Here's how to set up a partial-fill piggyback set: Begin the partial-fill piggyback procedure by following the steps for adding medication to a primary I.V. line. Swab the container. Read the medication's directions. If it needs to be reconstituted, refer back to page 62 to find out how. If it's ready for use, draw the medication into a syringe. Then, insert the needle into the partial-fill piggyback container and inject the medication.
- Label the piggyback bottle with the following information: the medication added, the date and time of addition, and your initials.
- Close the piggyback line flow clamp. Push the spike into the top of the piggyback bottle.
- Attach an 18G or 19G 1" needle to the piggyback line. (Don't use a needle over 1" long or you'll puncture the primary tubing.) Open the flow clamp for a few seconds to prime the piggyback tubing and needle. Then close it.
- Label the secondary tubing with the date and time you establish the line. Hang the set on the remaining I.V. pole hook.
- Swab the piggyback port of the primary I.V. line with alcohol. Make sure the medication you're admin-

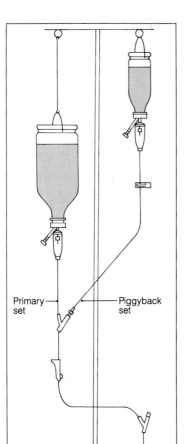

Primary set — Piggyback set

istering is compatible with the primary I.V. solution. If it's not, flush the primary I.V. line with saline solution before connecting the piggyback line. If it is compatible, insert the piggyback set needle into the piggyback port and tape it.
- Use the extension hook provided to rehang the primary container. Its center of gravity must be lower than the minibottle.
- Open the piggyback line flow clamp. Because the minibottle's placed higher, the backcheck valve will automatically cut off the flow of primary solution and allow the medication to flow. Adjust the flow to the medication's recommended rate.
- When the piggyback solution level drops below the drip chamber of the primary container, the bankcheck valve cuts off the piggyback flow. Then, the primary solution automatically begins running again.

### Using a secondary I.V. set

Here's the general procedure for establishing a secondary line: Begin by reading the medication package insert. If you need to reconstitute the medication, follow the steps on page 62. Then, use these instructions to proceed:
- Draw up the medication with a filter needle and syringe. Remember, a filter needle's good only once. Replace it immediately with a large-bore (18G) 1½" needle.
- Swab the secondary bottle stopper with alcohol. Then, inject the medication into the secondary bottle. Gently rotate it to mix the solution.
- Affix a *medication added* label to the container. Include drug dose; date and time; expiration date; patient's name, room and bed number, and your initials.
- Attach the tubing to the secondary bottle by driving the spike into the bottle stopper. Hang the set.

Note: Some medications now come in vials suitable for hanging directly on an I.V. pole. With this type, you don't have to prepare medication and inject it into a bottle. Instead, you can inject diluent directly into the medica-

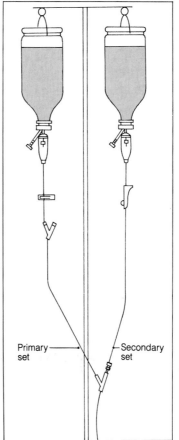

Primary set — Secondary set

tion vial. Then, spike the vial, prime the tubing, and hang the set as usual.
- Attach a 20G 1" needle to the tubing adapter. Prime the entire secondary set.

Make sure the medication's compatible with the primary line solution. If it isn't, swab the secondary port. Then, flush the primary tubing with saline solution before inserting the set's needle.
- If the medication's compatible, swab the secondary port and insert the 20G 1" needle. Use two 3" strips of ¼" tape to secure the needle in the port, as shown here.

Begin infusing the medication at the prescribed rate. Follow the doctor's orders; he may want it to run with the primary solution, or he may want it to run by itself. Document what you've done.

# Intravenous administration

### Troubleshooting I.V. therapy

To perform venipuncture successfully, you must place the needle squarely in the vein. One way you can confirm proper needle placement following insertion is by checking for blood backflow. What if you have problems getting a blood backflow? Then, read this chart. The tips it includes may help.

| Problem | Possible cause | Intervention |
|---|---|---|
| No blood backflow | Needle is pressed against the opposite wall of the vein | Pull the needle back slightly. |
| Slight blood backflow at first, then none | Needle has passed through the opposite wall of the vein | Withdraw needle and begin again. |
| Blood backflow present, but I.V. solution flow rate is sluggish | Needle is in the vein but pushed against a valve | Advance the needle slightly, and check for blood backflow again. |

If you're using the drip method, your greatest problem may be a sluggish flow rate. The cause could be obvious; for example, a drip chamber that's less than half full or a kinked tube. In other cases, the cause may be hidden. If you don't know why the flow rate's sluggish, try these solutions: Wrap the tubing around a pencil, and then quickly pull the pencil out of the coil. Or tape a 2" x 2" sterile gauze pad either over or under the catheter to change the catheter entry angle. For a more detailed look at troubleshooting problems you may encounter during I.V. therapy, see the NURSING PHOTOBOOK *Managing I.V. Therapy.*

### Avoiding common I.V. problems

The best way to avoid I.V. complications is to learn the proper procedures *before* starting therapy. Otherwise, you could be faced with a variety of problems. The four most common are detailed below. For more information on I.V. complications and how to avoid them, see the NURSING PHOTOBOOK *Managing I.V. Therapy.*

| Complication | Possible causes | Signs and symptoms | Nursing considerations | Prevention tips |
|---|---|---|---|---|
| **Infiltration** | • Needle displacement (either partial or complete)<br>• Leakage of blood around needle (especially likely in an older patient whose tissues have lost their elasticity) | • Coolness of skin around site<br>• Swelling around site<br>• Absence of blood backflow. If a tourniquet's applied above the site, the infusion continues to run.<br>• Sluggish flow rate | • Discontinue the infusion, and remove the needle immediately.<br>• If swelling's small, apply ice. Otherwise, apply warm wet compresses.<br>• Restart I.V. in another limb.<br>• Document what you've done. | • Use a splint to stabilize the needle or catheter when the site's over a joint or the patient's active.<br>• Palpate occasionally to confirm proper needle position. |
| **Thrombophlebitis** | • Injury to the vein, either during venipuncture or from needle movement later<br>• Irritation to the vein caused by the following: long-term therapy, irritating or incompatible additives, or use of a vein that's too small to handle the amount or type of solution.<br>• Sluggish flow rate, which allows a clot to form at the end of the needle or catheter | • Sluggish flow rate<br>• Edema in limb<br>• A vein that's sore, hard, cord-like, and warm to the touch. It may look like a red line above the venipuncture site. | • Discontinue the infusion, and remove the needle immediately.<br>• Apply warm wet compresses.<br>• Notify doctor.<br>• Restart I.V. in another limb.<br>• Document what you've done.<br>• *Important:* Never try to irrigate the line. In addition to increasing the risk of infection, you may flush a clot into the bloodstream, causing an embolus. | • If you have to use an irritating additive, try to find a vein large enough to dilute it. Dilute irritating additives with diluents, if possible.<br>• Make sure drug additives are compatible.<br>• Keep the infusion flowing at the prescribed rate.<br>• Stabilize the needle or catheter with a splint, if necessary. |
| **Systemic infection** (more common with plastic catheters than with metal needles) | • Poor aseptic technique<br>• Contamination of equipment during manufacture, storage, or use<br>• Irrigation of clogged I.V. | • Sudden rise in temperature and pulse<br>• Chills and shaking<br>• Blood pressure changes | • Look for other sources of infection first. Culture urine, sputum, and blood, as ordered.<br>• Discontinue the I.V. immediately. Send equipment to the lab for bacterial analysis.<br>• Restart I.V. in another limb.<br>• Document what you've done. | • Review and improve aseptic technique.<br>• Avoid contaminating the site when bathing the patient.<br>• If any parts of the system are accidentally disconnected, replace them with sterile equipment. |
| **Speed shock** | • Drugs administered too quickly<br>• Improper administration of bolus infusions | • Headache<br>• Tight feeling in chest<br>• Irregular pulse<br>• Shock, cardiac arrest | • Discontinue drug infusion.<br>• Begin infusing 5% dextrose in water at KVO rate.<br>• Notify doctor immediately.<br>• Document what you've done. | • Keep infusion flowing at prescribed rate. |

# Intra-arterial administration

Although you may never insert an arterial line, you *may* use one to deliver medications. Are you familiar with the basic functions of an arterial line? For example, do you know that it can be used for:
• taking a blood sample?
• taking blood pressure readings?
• infusing chemotherapeutic drugs directly into a malignant tumor?

On the next few pages, we'll be focusing on the last of these three uses. By infusing chemotherapeutic agents directly into a tumor, you deliver the maximum medication concentration to the malignant cells without causing systemic effects or destroying normal cells. To learn more about using arterial lines for medication delivery, read on.

## Selecting your equipment

As you know, any medication the doctor administers through an arterial line must be delivered under pressure. To meet this requirement, you'll need one of the three types of infusion equipment shown on this chart. Compare their advantages and disadvantages.

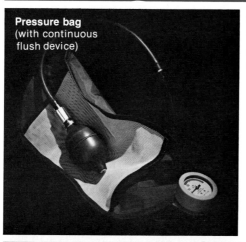

**Pressure bag** (with continuous flush device)

| Advantages | Disadvantages |
|---|---|
| • Inexpensive<br>• Easy to operate | • Not as accurate as an infusion pump<br>• Must be checked every half hour for pressure variations<br>• No alarm system |

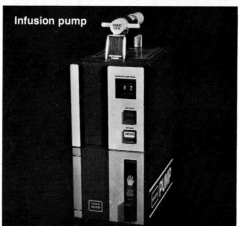

**Infusion pump**

| Advantages | Disadvantages |
|---|---|
| • Precise<br>• Provides useful information at a glance<br>• Has helpful safety features | • Expensive<br>• Takes time to set up<br>• Bulky<br>• Must be serviced by a company representative |

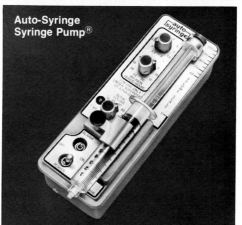

**Auto-Syringe Syringe Pump®**

| Advantages | Disadvantages |
|---|---|
| • Small and portable<br>• Precise<br>• Can be used at home<br>• Has helpful safety features | • Expensive<br>• Must be serviced by a company representative |

# Intra-arterial administration

**Preparing the patient for arterial line insertion**

Is your patient scheduled to receive chemotherapy through an arterial line? Take time to prepare him properly. Explain the procedure. Answer his questions honestly. If you can't, ask the doctor to discuss things further.

Make sure the patient's on a liquid diet at least *12 hours* before his arterial line is inserted. However, don't give anything orally if the insertion requires *major* surgery. Before insertion, record the color, temperature, and blanching time of the area around the intended site. This information will serve as baseline data you can use for comparison *after* insertion and during therapy.

The doctor begins the procedure by identifying the artery that supplies the tumor site. He'll then use fluoroscopy to insert a radiopaque catheter. In some cases, surgical insertion isn't necessary, because the doctor can use fluoroscopy to insert the catheter percutaneously. When it's possible, this method is preferred over surgical insertion, because it reduces the risk of hemorrhage and of arterial thrombosis.

After the doctor sutures the catheter in place, apply a sterile dressing.

## Managing an arterial line

Usually the doctor manages an arterial line, but in your hospital, you may be responsible for maintaining it. Here's how:

Check the fluid containers and tubing connections at least twice each shift, and replace them daily. When you replace the fluid container, add heparin to the prescribed medication (if your hospital's policy calls for it). Check the doctor's order to determine the exact proportions.

Because of strong arterial blood pressure, all fluids must be infused with either a pump or a pressure bag Check the infusion equipment periodically. Maintain the correct flow rate, or the line may become occluded. Change the dressing on the site at least three times a week.

## Changing an arterial line dressing

**1** Whenever you change the dressing on an arterial line, you must use aseptic technique. Begin by removing the old dressing and dispose of it correctly. Then, put on sterile gloves and inspect the site for signs of infection; for example, redness, heat, pain, swelling, or purulent discharge. If you observe any, or your patient has a fever, call the doctor.

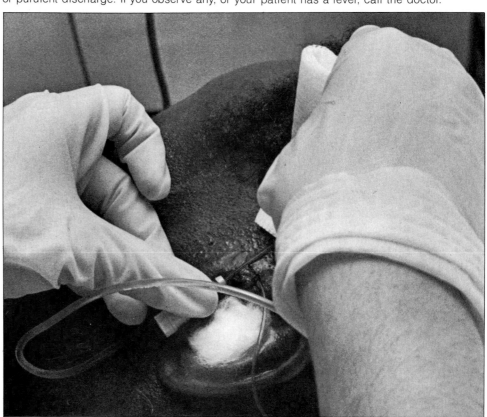

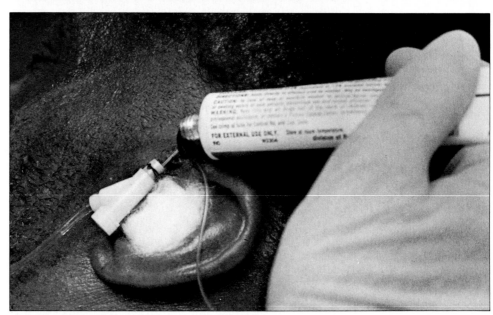

**2** Now, swab the site with antiseptic solution, beginning at the center and working outward in a circular pattern. Clean an area 3″ to 4″ (7.6 to 10 cm) in diameter. Then, apply antimicrobial ointment around the site, as shown in this photo.

COMPLICATIONS

**3** Finally, cover the site with several occlusive sterile gauze pads. Tape them in place, making sure you don't kink the tubing in the process.

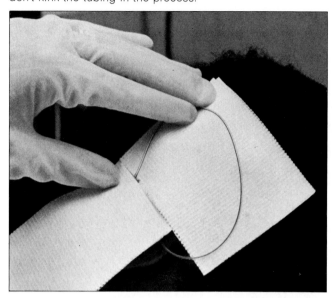

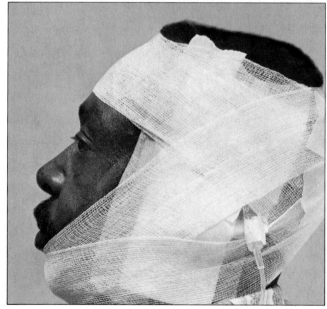

**4** Make sure the dressing is secure, as shown in this photo. Once each hour, document the color, temperature, and blanching time of the area around the site. If you notice any significant change, notify the doctor.

Also check the patient's arterial pulse distal to insertion site. Document your findings, as follows: once each hour for the first 24 hours; then, once every 2 to 4 hours for the second 24 hours; and finally, once every 8 hours until instructed otherwise.

When the therapy's discontinued, the doctor will remove the line and apply a pressure bandage to the site. Examine the site every hour for the first 24 hours afterward, and tell the doctor if you see signs of a hematoma.

### When the patient has an arterial line: Coping with problems

| Signs and symptoms | Possible cause | Intervention |
|---|---|---|
| Twitching, paresthesia, motor weakness | Improper catheter placement | Notify doctor. He'll reposition the catheter tip. |
| Vasospasm, arteritis | Foreign bodies in medication or catheter | Notify doctor. He'll order appropriate therapy; for example, an anesthetic, like lidocaine hydrochloride (Xylocaine*), for vasospasm; or an anti-inflammatory drug for arteritis. |
| Pain or numbness in extremity; or severe visceral pain | Clotting in catheter | Notify doctor. He may replace the catheter. If therapy is interrupted, the doctor will probably order dilute heparin injected into the catheter to prevent clotting. |
| Swelling, bleeding around site | Internal bleeding from heparin accumulation around site | Notify doctor. Apply external pressure and warm, moist heat to the site. Follow aseptic dressing technique. |
| Dilated blood vessels (as determined by X-ray) | Weakened vessel wall from catheter pressure | Notify doctor. He'll probably remove the catheter to prevent hemorrhaging. |
| Local swelling, drainage at insertion site | Infection from fluid or equipment contamination; infrequent dressing changes; lack of aseptic technique | Notify doctor. He may remove the line or order application of antibiotic ointment to the site, and systemic antibiotics. |
| Labored breathing, respiratory collapse | Air embolism, or air bubbles in line, caused by a disconnection or an empty infusion bottle | Notify doctor. Place the patient on his left side, in the Trendelenburg position. This will encourage the embolism to travel to the right atrium of the heart, where, hopefully, it'll be absorbed. |

*Available in the United States and in Canada.

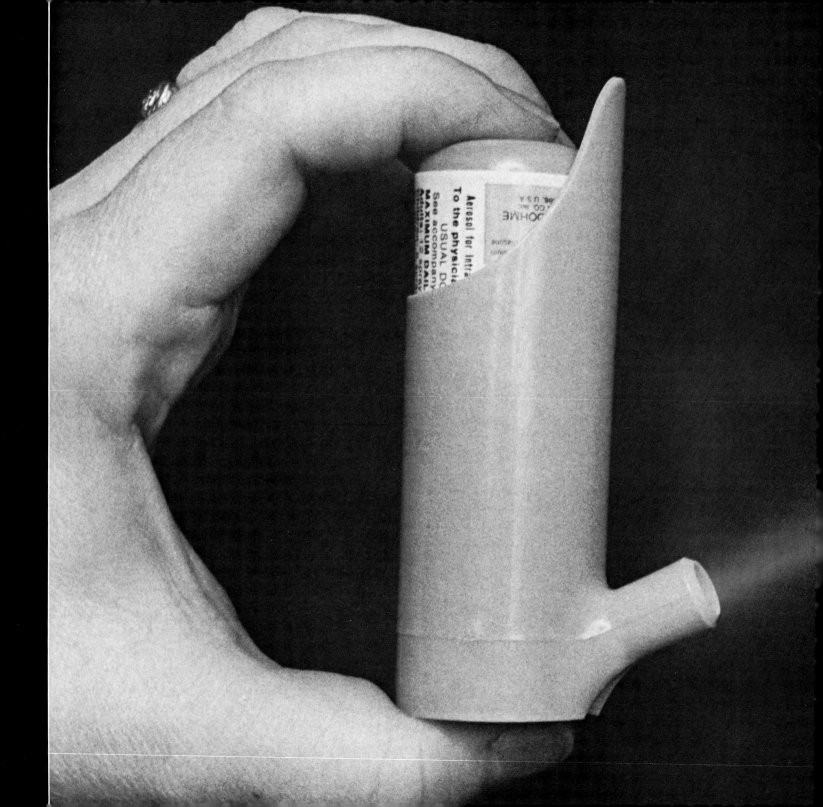

# Administering by the Respiratory Route

Instillation

Inhalation

# Instillation

You probably know what nasal instillation is: the process of administering liquid medication in the patient's nose, either in drop form or as a spray. But do you know the best techniques for instilling medication? For example, do you know:
• how to position the patient for maxillary sinus treatment?
• how to safely instill drops in an infant?
• how to use an atomizer or nasal aerosol device correctly?

If you're not sure, read the following pages.

## Understanding your patient's upper respiratory tract

Before you instill any nasal medication, review your knowledge of the upper respiratory tract. To jog your memory, take a look at the illustrations on these pages.

As you can see in the illustration at the right, the nose is divided by the septum into two chambers called nares, or nostrils. The nasal passages connect four pairs of nasal sinuses: ethmoidal, sphenoidal, maxillary, and frontal.

The respiratory tract is lined with ciliated columnar epithelium which, in turn, is covered with an acidic layer of mucus produced by the goblet cells (see the illustration below). Normally, this mucous layer captures most inhaled dirt and bacteria.

Then, propelled by the cilia, it carries the contaminants to the nasopharynx, where they're expelled.

But suppose the acidic environment of the nasal cavity is disturbed by infection, allergy, trauma, sudden temperature change, or irritating gases or particles. In such cases, ciliary movement slows or stops altogether. The mucous membrane swells and becomes congested with mucus and contaminants. And this, of course, makes breathing difficult and uncomfortable.

When you teach your patient how to instill nasal medication himself, show and explain these illustrations. They'll help him understand how his upper respiratory tract works.

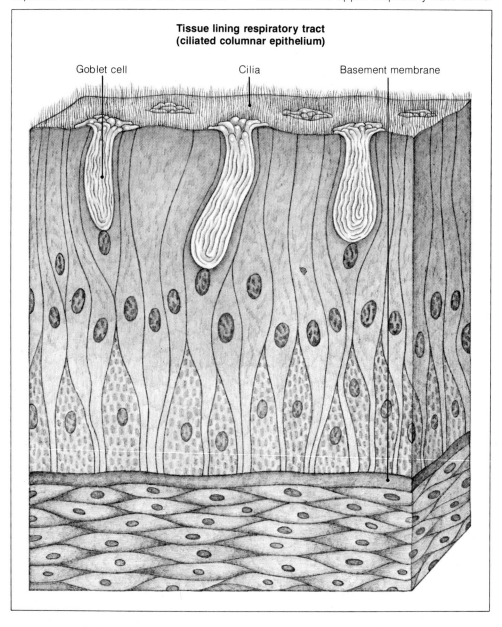

**Tissue lining respiratory tract
(ciliated columnar epithelium)**

Goblet cell          Cilia          Basement membrane

**Upper airway anatomy**

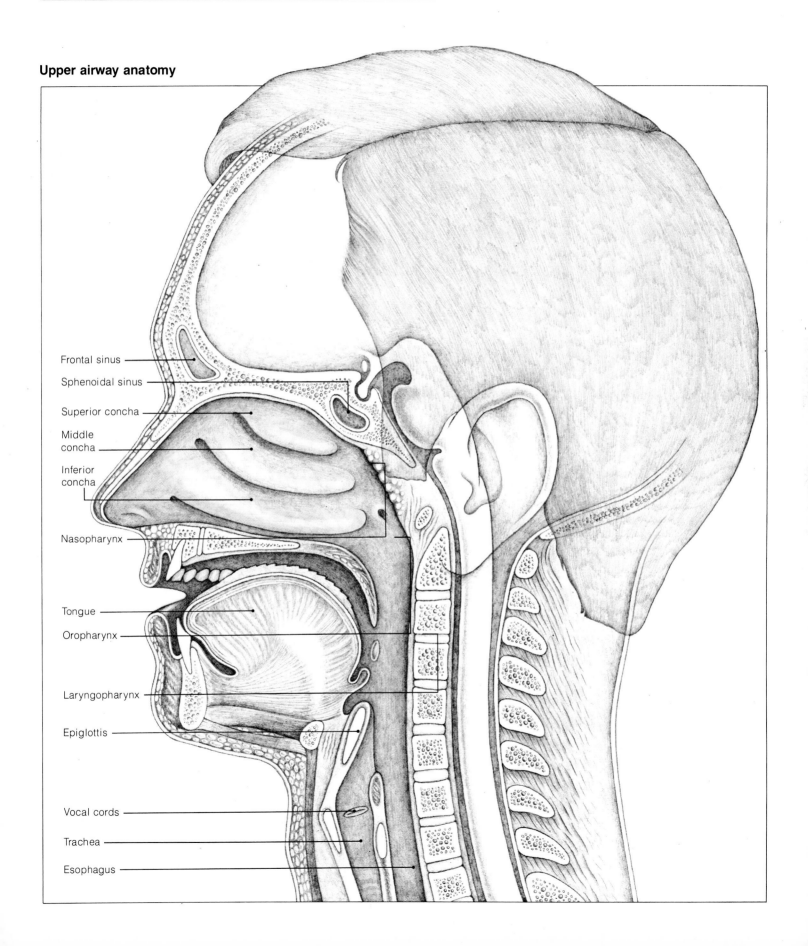

Frontal sinus

Sphenoidal sinus

Superior concha

Middle concha

Inferior concha

Nasopharynx

Tongue

Oropharynx

Laryngopharynx

Epiglottis

Vocal cords

Trachea

Esophagus

# Instillation

## Learning about nasal medications

Most of the nasal medications you'll give by instillation act as vasoconstricting (sympathomimetic) agents, which coat and shrink swollen mucous membranes. Others are antiseptics or local anesthetics. But all of them produce local, rather than systemic, effects in the patient's upper respiratory tract. To instill them, use a dropper or an atomizer (which produces a spray).

Nasal medications are usually aqueous, isotonic, slightly acidic, and nonirritating. But they're never oily. Why? Because an oily medication would inhibit ciliary activity and increase the risk of respiratory infection. What's more, if the patient inhaled an oily medication, he could develop lipoid pneumonia.

## Positioning the patient to treat her sinuses

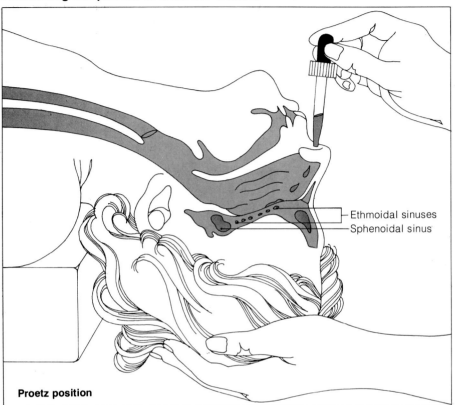

Proetz position

Ethmoidal sinuses
Sphenoidal sinus

**1** *Your patient has a sinus condition for which the doctor's ordered nose drops. Do you know how to position the patient correctly? If you're not sure, study these illustrations.*

To instill medication in both the ethmoidal and the sphenoidal sinuses, place your patient in the Proetz position, shown here. Put her on her back, with her shoulders elevated and her head tilted back.

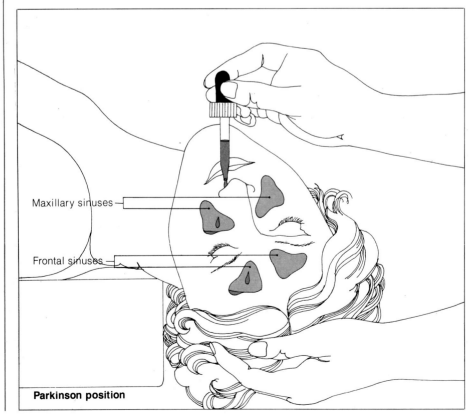

Maxillary sinuses

Frontal sinuses

Parkinson position

**2** Use the Parkinson position to treat the maxillary and the frontal sinuses, located on each side of her face. As you can see here, this position is like the Proetz position, except the patient's head is tilted to one side instead of straight back.

*Important:* No matter which position you use, take care not to contaminate the dropper by touching the nostrils.

### Giving nose drops to an adult

**1** *Is your patient's nose congested? If the doctor orders, you can make her more comfortable by administering nose drops. Just follow these steps, remembering to maintain clean technique throughout the procedure.*

First, confirm the order, and assemble the equipment you see here: the bottle of medication, a medicine dropper, and tissues. Wash your hands, and explain the procedure to the patient. Remember to warn her that she may taste the drops.

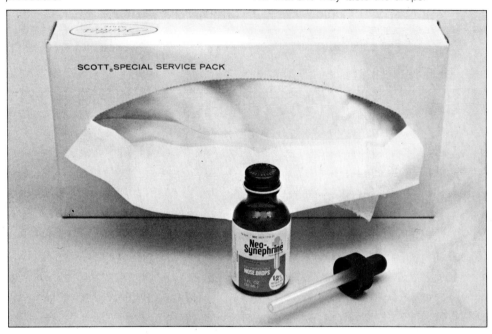

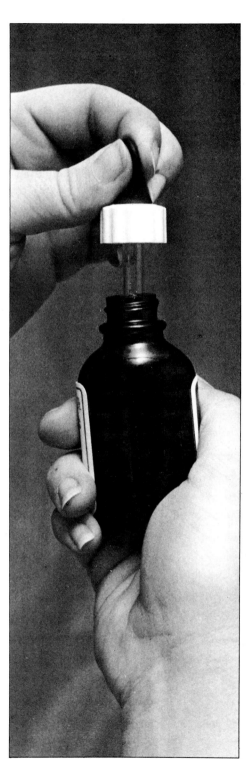

**2** How should you position the patient? If your patient has a sinus condition, place her in either the Proetz position or the Parkinson position, as illustrated on the opposite page. However, if your patient suffers from ordinary nasal congestion, as does the one shown here, seat her upright, with room to tilt her head back. *Note:* If she's *unable* to sit up, place her in the Proetz position.

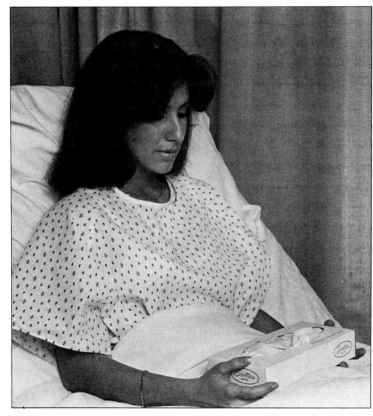

**3** Now, draw enough medication into the dropper to instill the prescribed number of drops into the patient's nostrils. Otherwise, you'll have to reinsert the dropper into the bottle, increasing the risk of contamination.

# Instillation

**Giving nose drops to an adult** continued

**4** Open the patient's nostril completely, by pushing up gently on the tip of her nose. Place the dropper about ⅓" (1 cm) inside the nostril. To minimize the risk of contaminating the dropper, take care not to let it touch your patient's nose.

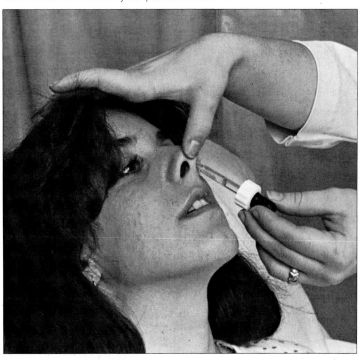

**6** Take care to prevent the patient from aspirating any medication. If she coughs, seat her upright and pat her back. Then, observe her closely for several minutes to see if any further respiratory problems develop.

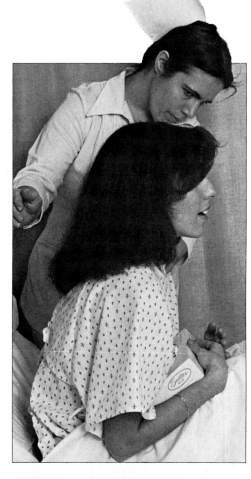

**5** Now, direct the tip of the dropper toward the midline of the superior concha, as shown in this illustration. This position will permit the medication to flow down the back of the patient's nose, not her throat.

Squeeze the dropper bulb to instill the correct number of drops into the nostril. Repeat the process in the other nostril, if ordered.

*Important:* As you're instilling the drops, ask the patient to breathe through her mouth. This will suppress her urge to sniff, which could propel medication into her sinuses.

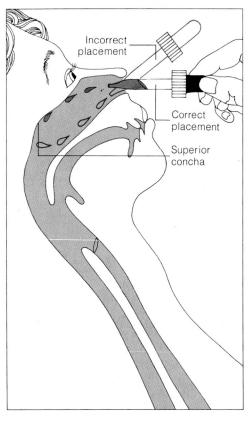

Incorrect placement

Correct placement

Superior concha

**7** When you've instilled the correct number of drops, tell your patient to keep her head tilted back for about 5 minutes. But allow her to expectorate any medication that runs into her throat, since it may have an unpleasant taste. Provide her with tissues. Finally, document the entire procedure in your nurses' notes.

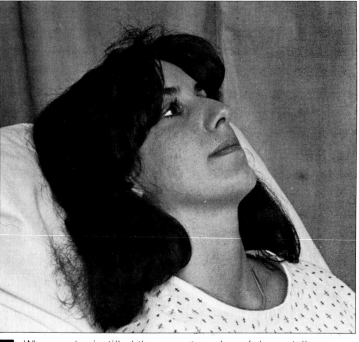

## Giving nose drops to an infant

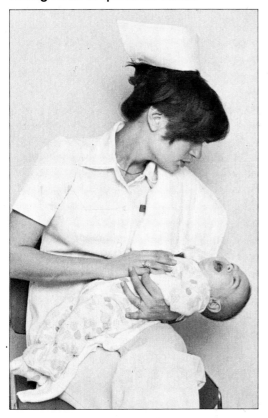

**1** *Under normal circumstances, an infant usually breathes through his nose. So if you're caring for an infant with nasal congestion, he'll have difficulty sucking. To relieve the problem, the doctor will probably want you to administer nose drops 20 to 30 minutes before each feeding. Here's how:*

First, check the medication order against the Kardex. Then, wash your hands and gather the following equipment: the bottle of medication, a medication dropper, and tissues. Choose a dropper with a protective rubber tip.

*Important:* Warm the medication by running warm water over the bottle for several minutes. Or warm it by carrying the bottle in your pocket for 30 minutes before you administer the medication.

Now, carefully position the infant so his head is tilted back on your arm, as shown here.

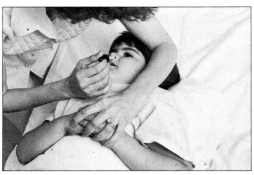

**2** Suppose your patient is a child? If she's too large to hold in your arms, place her on her back, with a small pillow under her shoulders. Gently tilt back her head, supporting it between your forearm and your body, as shown here. Use one of your hands to restrain her arms and hands.

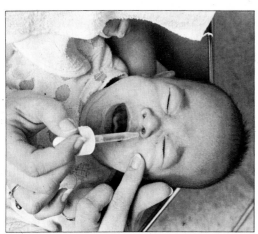

**3** Draw the medication into the dropper. If possible, open the infant's nostrils by gently pushing up the tip of his nose. Instill the ordered number of drops in the nostril. Avoid touching the nostril with the dropper.

Repeat the process in the other nostril, if ordered.

After instilling the drops, keep the infant's head tilted back for 3 to 5 minutes (if possible). Stay alert for any sign of aspiration. If he begins to cough, sit him upright and pat his back until he's cleared his lungs.

*Important:* If he's aspirated a large amount of medication, clear his respiratory tract with nasotracheal suctioning.

Finally, document the entire procedure and the infant's response.

**Teaching the patient about nose drops**

Your patient's about to be discharged. If the doctor's prescribed nose drops for him to use at home, show him how to instill them properly. Be sure he knows the name of his medication and the prescribed dosage. In addition:
• Urge your patient to follow the doctor's orders exactly, and explain the dangers of overusing the medication.
• Because nose drops are easily contaminated, advise your patient not to buy more than he'll use in a short time. Instruct him to discard the medication if it has sediment or looks discolored.
• Warn your patient not to share his medication with family members. Doing so may spread infection.
• Tell him to call the doctor if he notices any side effects.

**Teaching the patient about nasal sprays**

Does your patient need nasal spray delivered by atomizer or a nasal aerosol device? Teach him how to administer it, using one of the home care aids on the next two pages. As examples, we've featured Turbinaire Decadron Phosphate (a nasal aerosol) and a common hand-held atomizer. (For more information about Turbinaire Decadron Phosphate, turn to the chart on page 110.)

*Note:* If your patient's using an atomizer, teach him how to use it the very first administration. *You* may squeeze the atomizer too hard, propelling the spray into your patient's sinuses and eustachian tubes. (If the patient can't do the procedure himself, ask the doctor to order nose drops instead.)

# Patient teaching

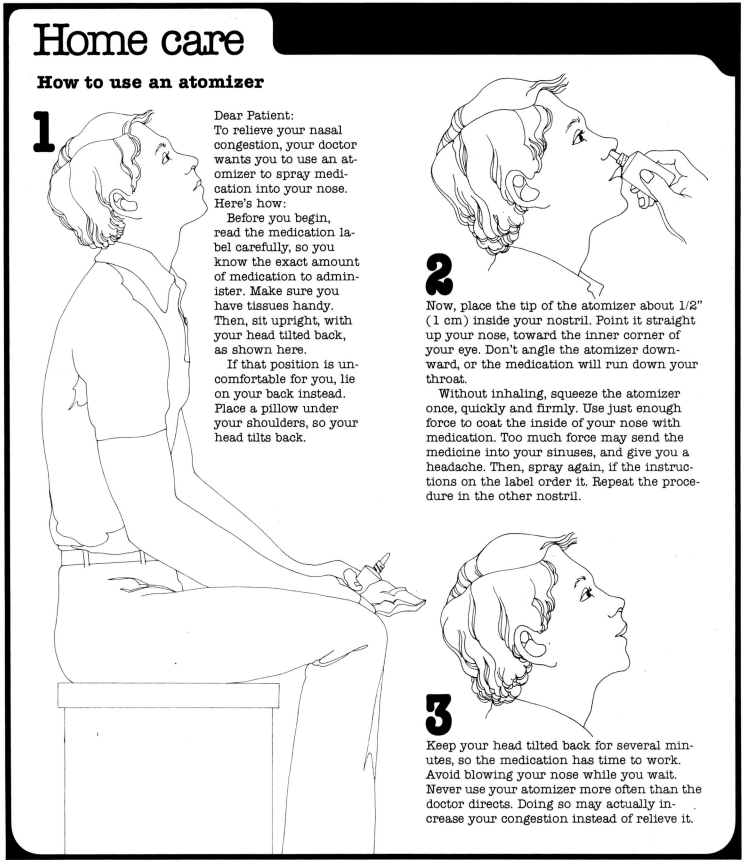

# Home care

## How to use an atomizer

**1**

Dear Patient:
To relieve your nasal congestion, your doctor wants you to use an atomizer to spray medication into your nose. Here's how:

Before you begin, read the medication label carefully, so you know the exact amount of medication to administer. Make sure you have tissues handy. Then, sit upright, with your head tilted back, as shown here.

If that position is uncomfortable for you, lie on your back instead. Place a pillow under your shoulders, so your head tilts back.

**2**

Now, place the tip of the atomizer about 1/2" (1 cm) inside your nostril. Point it straight up your nose, toward the inner corner of your eye. Don't angle the atomizer downward, or the medication will run down your throat.

Without inhaling, squeeze the atomizer once, quickly and firmly. Use just enough force to coat the inside of your nose with medication. Too much force may send the medicine into your sinuses, and give you a headache. Then, spray again, if the instructions on the label order it. Repeat the procedure in the other nostril.

**3**

Keep your head tilted back for several minutes, so the medication has time to work. Avoid blowing your nose while you wait. Never use your atomizer more often than the doctor directs. Doing so may actually increase your congestion instead of relieve it.

# Home care

## How to use a nasal aerosol device (Turbinaire®)

**1**

Dear Patient:
Your doctor wants you to use a medicated aerosol spray to relieve nasal irritation. Here's how: First, read the medication label so you know the exact amount of medication to administer. Then, put together the spray device by placing the stem of the medication cartridge in the plastic nasal adapter, as shown here. (If you're inserting a refill cartridge, first remove the protective cap from the stem.)

**2**

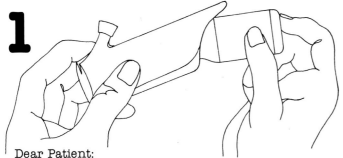

Now, gently blow your nose to remove excess mucus.

**3**

Shake the device well. Remove the protective cap from the adapter tip.

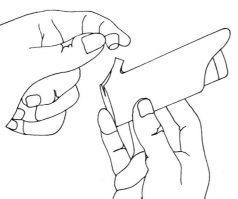

**4**

Now, place the tip inside your nostril. Holding your breath, firmly press down once on the cartridge; then, release it. Continue to hold your breath for several seconds afterward. Don't inhale the mist.

**5**

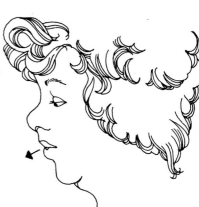

Remove the adapter tip from your nostril and exhale. If necessary, reinsert the adapter in the same nostril, and spray again. Then, repeat this procedure in the other nostril, if ordered. Important: Don't blow your nose for at least 2 minutes.

**6**

Replace the protective cap on the adapter tip. Then, put the entire device in a plastic bag, to keep it clean. Once a day, remove the medication cartridge and thoroughly rinse the plastic adapter with warm water.

   Caution: Follow the doctor's directions exactly. Let him know at once if you feel increased nasal irritation, itching, or bleeding; increased nasal congestion; coughing; headache; or dizziness.

# Inhalation

How much do you know about inhalation therapy? If you're caring for an asthma patient, he probably has a hand-held nebulizer to deliver bronchial medication.

But can you be sure he's using it properly? If he's not, he may not get the maximum benefit from the medication. What's worse, he could suffer serious side effects from overuse. On the following pages, you'll learn what to tell him about the safe, effective use of nebulizers.

And that's not all you'll learn about inhalation therapy. Do you know how to set up a vaporizer? What complications to watch for during IPPB therapy? And how about oxygen therapy? Can you recognize the danger signs of respiratory depression or of atelectasis? If you're not sure, this section will help you.

## How inhalation therapy works

When you administer inhalation therapy to your patient, you introduce one or more of the following drug forms into his lower respiratory tract: a gaseous drug, like oxygen; a vaporized or nebulized liquid drug; or a finely powdered solid drug. Most of these drugs, like mucolytics and bronchodilators, are given for local effects. A few, like oxygen, are given for systemic effects. But remember, *any* drug your patient inhales may produce unintended systemic effects because of the lungs' great capacity to absorb drugs directly into the bloodstream.

How deeply does inhaled medication penetrate the lower respiratory tract? This may vary, depending on the patient's depth of inspiration, his degree of congestion, and the size of the drug particles. But in most cases, you'll find that the smaller the particles, the deeper their penetration.

Study this illustration. As you can see, when drug particles between 10 and 40 microns are inhaled, they're deposited in the patient's upper airway. Those between 3 and 10 microns are deposited in the bronchi, and those 1 or 2 microns are deposited in the deepest recesses of the lungs. But particles smaller than 1 micron aren't deposited at all; they're exhaled.

## Giving inhalation therapy: Advantages and disadvantages

*Is the doctor considering inhalation therapy for your patient? Before he makes a decision, he'll consider these points:*

### Advantages
• The lungs' large surface area and rich capillary network allow fast drug absorption and distribution. Only the intravenous route achieves higher blood levels of a drug more quickly than the respiratory route.
• Potent drugs may be given in small doses, minimizing their side effects.
• The respiratory route's easily accessible, providing a convenient alternative when other routes are unavailable.

### Disadvantages
• Dosage accuracy's difficult to achieve.
• The patient must be able to cooperate by breathing deeply as therapy's given (unless he's mechanically ventilated).
• The patient may gag on unpleasant-tasting medication.
• The patient's trachea or bronchi may become irritated, causing coughing or bronchospasm.
• An asthmatic patient may become dependent on a hand-held nebulizer.
• When not kept clean, hand-held nebulizers are a source of infection.

## Drug absorption in an alveolus

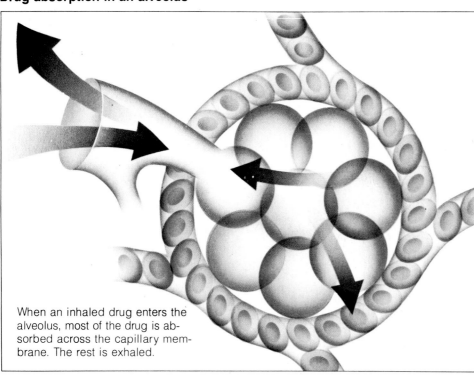

When an inhaled drug enters the alveolus, most of the drug is absorbed across the capillary membrane. The rest is exhaled.

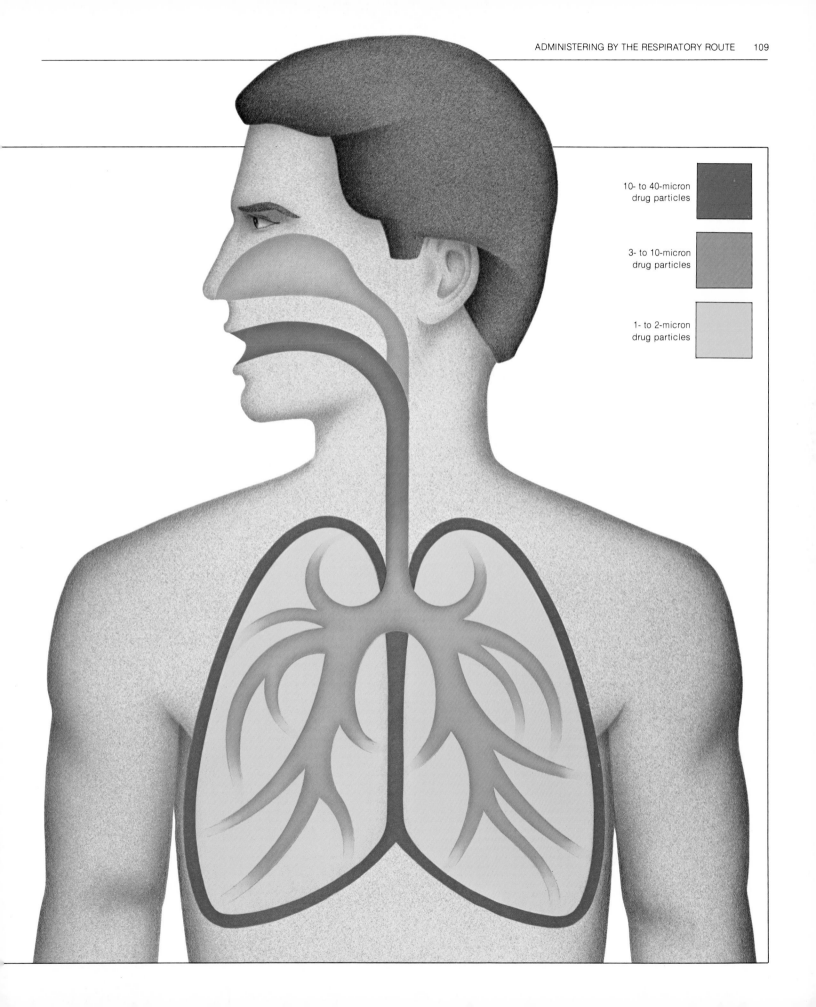

10- to 40-micron
drug particles

3- to 10-micron
drug particles

1- to 2-micron
drug particles

# Inhalation

## Nurses' guide to aerosol therapy drugs

| Drug | Indications and dosage | Side effects |
|------|------------------------|--------------|
| **epinephrine 1:1,000** Adrenalin*, Medihaler-Epi*, Primatene Mist, Vaponefrin* | *For use as a bronchodilator:* **Adults:** 0.2 mg per dose. One to two inhalations, as needed. Do not administer more than three inhalation treatments per day. | Blood pressure changes, tachycardia, excitement, tremor. May also cause angina when coronary insufficiency is present. |
| **isoproterenol hydrochloride** Isuprel*, Medihaler-Iso* | *For use as a bronchodilator:* **Adults:** 0.5 ml of 1:200 solution in 2 to 2.5 ml normal saline solution inhaled over 15 minutes. One to two inhalations four to six times daily. Do not administer more than six inhalations per day. | Hypotension, tachycardia, nausea, headache, flushing, palpitations; parotid swelling (with prolonged use) |
| **isoetharine** Bronkometer, Bronkosol | *For use as a bronchodilator:* **Adults:** 0.25 to 1 ml diluted 1:3 with saline solution and administered IPPB over 10 to 15 minutes once every 4 hours. When given with hand-held nebulizer, three to seven inhalations undiluted every 4 hours. When given with aerosol nebulizer, one to two inhalations, as needed. | Blood pressure changes, palpitations, nausea, tachycardia |
| **metaproterenol sulfate** Alupent*, Metaprel | *For use as a bronchodilator:* **Adults and children (over age 12):** Two to three inhalations every 3 to 4 hours, as needed. Do not administer more than 12 inhalations per day. | Nervousness, weakness, drowsiness, tremors, tachycardia, hypertension, palpitations, vomiting, nausea, bad taste; possible cardiac arrest (with excessive use) |
| **tyloxapol** Alevaire* | *For use as a mucolytic or as vehicle to deliver bronchodilators (isoproterenol, epinephrine, or phenylephrine):* **Adults:** 10 to 20 ml 0.125% solution administered by IPPB, given over 30 to 90 minutes, three to four times daily. Or 500 ml 0.125% solution administered by continuous aerosol over 12 to 24 hours. | Nausea |
| **acetylcysteine** Airbron**, Mucomyst*, NAC** | *For use as a mucolytic:* **Adults and children:** 1 to 2 ml 10% to 20% solution by direct instillation into trachea. Or 3 to 5 ml 20% solution inhaled three to four times daily. Or 6 to 10 ml 10% solution inhaled three to four times daily. In croupette: Up to 300 ml daily. | Rhinorrhea, hemoptysis, stomatitis, nausea, bronchospasm (mainly in asthmatics) |
| **dexamethasone sodium phosphate** Decadron Phosphate Respihaler, Turbinaire Decadron Phosphate | *A corticosteroid used to treat nasal polyps or bronchial asthma:* **Adults:** *Respihaler:* Three inhalations three to four times daily. Do not administer more than 12 inhalations daily. *Turbinaire:* Two sprays in each nostril two to three times daily. | Laryngeal or pharyngeal fungal infections, throat irritation, hoarseness, and coughing |
| **beclomethasone dipropionate** Vanceril* | *A corticosteroid used to treat bronchial asthma:* **Adults:** 100 mcg total given in two inhalations three to four times daily. Don't administer more than 20 inhalations daily. **Children (ages 6 thru 12):** One or two inhalations three to four times daily. Do not administer more than 10 inhalations daily. | Hoarseness, dry mouth; death from adrenal insufficiency during and after transfer from systemic steroids to beclomethasone |
| **cromolyn sodium** Intal* | *Used in combination with other drugs to treat patients with bronchial asthma:* **Adults and children (over age 2):** 20 mg inhaled four times daily by turbo-inhaler (Spinhaler) at regular intervals. | Bronchospasm, cough, nasal congestion, wheezing, angioedema, dizziness, dysuria, joint swelling, lacrimation, headache, nausea, rash, urticaria, swelling of parotid gland |

*Available both in the United States and Canada.
**Available only in Canada.

## Nursing considerations

- Monitor vital signs closely.
- Don't use if solution is brown or contains precipitate.
- Tell patient to wait 1 to 2 minutes between inhalations.
- Have patient rinse mouth after each treatment to prevent oropharynx dryness.
- Don't use concurrently with isoproterenol, although you may give these two drugs alternately.

- Monitor vital signs closely.
- Don't use if solution is brown or contains precipitate.
- Don't give concurrently with epinephrine.
- Have patient rinse mouth after each treatment. Instruct him not to swallow medicine or rinse water.
- Tell patient that sputum and saliva may be pink for awhile after inhalation.

- Monitor vital signs closely.
- Don't give concurrently with epinephrine.
- Teach patient how to use a metered-dose unit. (For details about the Bronkometer, see page 114.)
- Tell patient using aerosol nebulizer to wait 1 minute after first dose before repeating.

- Use with extreme caution in patients with hypertension, coronary artery disease, hyperthyroidism, or diabetes.
- Teach patient how to use metered-dose unit.
- Tell patient to call doctor if he does not respond to usual dose.
- Protect drug from light.

- Don't give with chlortetracycline.
- When used as vehicle, add bronchodilators just before use.
- Monitor and document cough (type and frequency).
- Urge patient not to smoke.

- Use with caution in asthmatics, elderly or debilitated patients.

- Use nonreactive metal, plastic, or glass when you administer by nebulization.
- Store drug in refrigerator after opening, and use within 96 hours.
- Monitor and document cough (type and frequency).
- Urge patient not to smoke.
- Don't mix with antibiotics.

- Instruct patient how to use device properly. (For tips on using the Turbinaire, see the home care aid on page 107.)
- Check patient's mouth for signs of fungal infection. Send culture to lab, if necessary.

- Contraindicated as a primary treatment for status asthmaticus.
- Check patient's mouth for signs of fungal infections. Send culture to lab, if necessary.
- Instruct patient how to use inhaler properly.

- Instruct patient how to use turbo-inhaler properly. (See the home care aid on pages 112 to 113.)
- If improvement occurs, it'll occur within 4 weeks.
- Discontinue if eosinophilic pneumonia occurs.
- Don't use for emergency treatment.
- Sudden discontinuation of this drug may necessitate reintroduction of oral corticosteroids.

### Teaching your patient how to use an inhalation device

The home care aids on the following pages will help you show your patient how to use an inhalation device properly. As examples, we've featured a whirlybird turbo-inhaler (Spinhaler®) and a metered-dose nebulizer (Bronkometer).

To begin, find a quiet area where you can work with your patient without being disturbed. Explain the procedure in terms he can understand, and go through it with him step by step. Then, have him demonstrate the procedure for you. Remember to encourage him to ask questions. Then answer them completely.

Make sure he knows:

- the name of the drug and its intended effects.

- the dosage, including how often to use it each day.

- the drug's potential side effects. For example, warn him to call his doctor if he develops palpitations, tremors, dizziness, or nausea.

- the procedure for assembling and cleaning the device. Stress the importance of keeping it clean. Remember, a hand-held nebulizer is especially prone to contamination.

In addition, emphasize the danger of abusing the drug; for example, dependence and overdose. Caution him not to use over-the-counter drugs in addition to his prescribed drug, because they may be incompatible. Tell him to notify his doctor if the prescribed drug seems ineffective. The doctor may adjust the prescription.

Finally, give him a copy of the appropriate home care aid, and review the instructions with him. For details on using other nebulizers, including the mininebulizer, see the NURSING PHOTOBOOK *Providing Respiratory Care.* For more information about the Spinhaler and the Bronkometer, see the chart on the opposite page.

# Patient teaching

## Home care

### How to use a turbo-inhaler

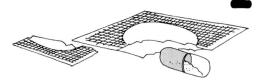

**1**
Dear Patient:
Inhaling the medication in this whirlybird inhalation device will help prevent asthma attacks. Use it exactly as your doctor ordered at these times: _____

Caution: Never use more than four capsules a day. Before you begin, wash and dry your hands. Unwrap one capsule so it's ready to use.

**2**
Then, hold the device so the white mouthpiece is on the bottom, like this. Slide the gray sleeve all the way to the top.

**4**
Firmly press the colored end of your medication capsule into the center of the propeller, as shown here. Avoid overhandling the capsule, or it may soften.

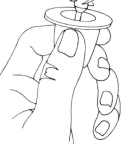

**3**
Open the mouthpiece by unscrewing its tip counterclockwise. Inside, you'll see a small propeller on a stem.

**5**
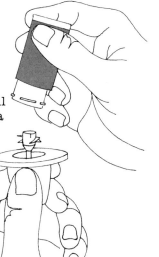
Now, screw the device back together securely, and hold it with the mouthpiece at the bottom, as shown here. To puncture the capsule and release the medication, slide the gray sleeve all the way down. Then, slide it up again. Do this step one time only.

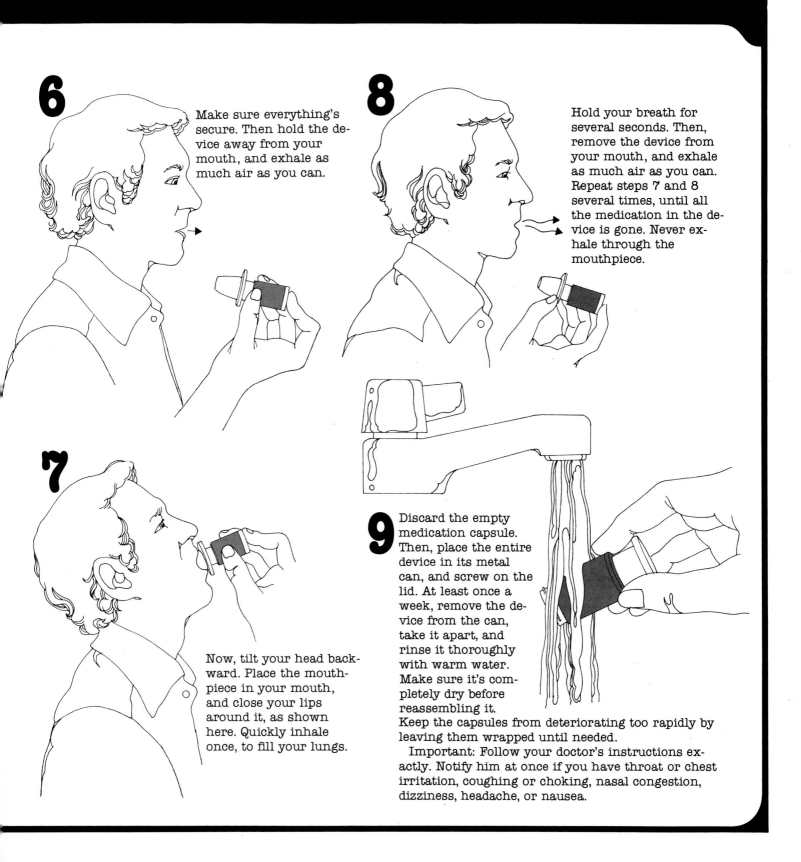

**6**
Make sure everything's secure. Then hold the device away from your mouth, and exhale as much air as you can.

**7**
Now, tilt your head backward. Place the mouthpiece in your mouth, and close your lips around it, as shown here. Quickly inhale once, to fill your lungs.

**8**
Hold your breath for several seconds. Then, remove the device from your mouth, and exhale as much air as you can. Repeat steps 7 and 8 several times, until all the medication in the device is gone. Never exhale through the mouthpiece.

**9**
Discard the empty medication capsule. Then, place the entire device in its metal can, and screw on the lid. At least once a week, remove the device from the can, take it apart, and rinse it thoroughly with warm water. Make sure it's completely dry before reassembling it.
Keep the capsules from deteriorating too rapidly by leaving them wrapped until needed.

Important: Follow your doctor's instructions exactly. Notify him at once if you have throat or chest irritation, coughing or choking, nasal congestion, dizziness, headache, or nausea.

# Patient teaching

## Home care

### How to use a metered-dose nebulizer

**1** Dear Patient:
Inhaling the medication in this metered-dose nebulizer will help you breathe more easily. Use it exactly as your doctor ordered at these times: _____
Here's how: First, remove the white mouthpiece and cap from the bottle. Then, remove the cap from the mouthpiece.

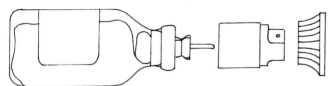

**2**
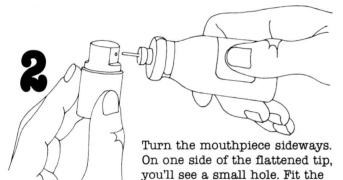
Turn the mouthpiece sideways. On one side of the flattened tip, you'll see a small hole. Fit the metal stem on the bottle into the hole.

**3**
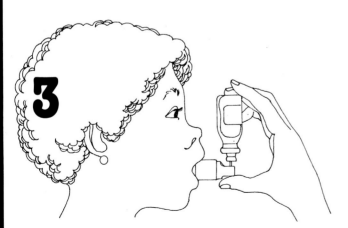
Now, exhale. Hold the nebulizer upside down, as you see here, and close your lips loosely around the mouthpiece.

**4**
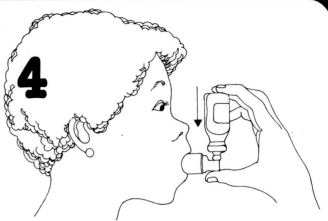
Inhale slowly. As you do, firmly push the bottle against the mouthpiece—one time only—to release one dose of medication. Continue inhaling until your lungs feel full.

**5**
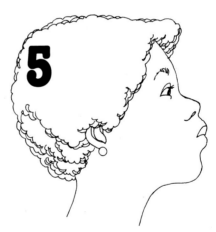
Take the mouthpiece away from your mouth, and hold your breath momentarily.

**6**
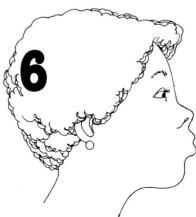
Then, purse your lips and exhale slowly. If the doctor directs, repeat the procedure. Important: Never overuse your nebulizer. Follow your doctor's instructions exactly. Finally, rinse the mouthpiece with warm water.

# Inhalation

## Using a vaporizer

**1** *If your patient suffers from nasal or bronchial congestion, use a vaporizer containing a medication like camphor or eucalyptus to make him more comfortable. Here's how to assemble it:*

After confirming the doctor's order, assemble the equipment: a vaporizer, the correct dose of prescribed medication, and 1,000 ml distilled water (with a ½ teaspoon of salt added). Explain the treatment to the patient.

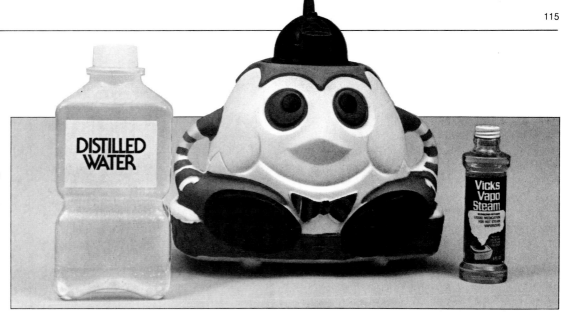

**2** Plug in the vaporizer. Then, pour in the distilled water until it reaches the level marked on the unit.

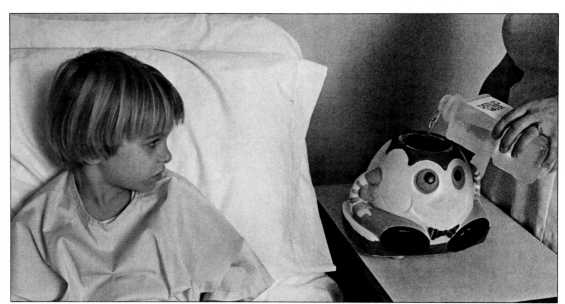

**3** Now, add the medication either to the water or to the cup at the top of the vaporizer (check the medication label for instructions). When the water vaporizes, the steam will diffuse the medication into the air.

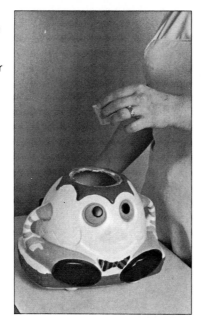

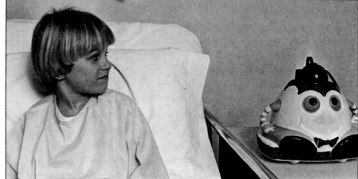

**4** Position the patient so he's comfortable. Put the vaporizer within several feet of him, so he can inhale the medicated steam easily. But don't put it so close that the steam burns him. For safety, place it on a chair or table, so no one trips over it.

Make sure the unit's working properly. Then document the procedure in your notes.

Check your patient's bed linen periodically. If it's damp, you've probably placed the vaporizer too close. Reposition it, and replace the bed linen.

# Inhalation

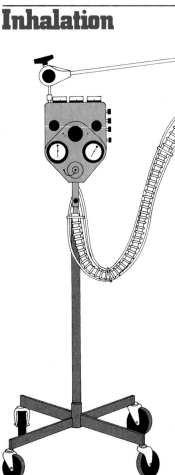

### What's IPPB therapy?

Consider the patient who needs prolonged nebulization therapy several times a day. To help him, the doctor may order intermittent positive pressure breathing (IPPB) therapy. Briefly, here's how it works:

First, set the ventilator for the prescribed pressure. Connect either a mouthpiece or a mask to the ventilator, and ask the patient to inhale through it. The ventilator will automatically force a flow of nebulized medication into the patient's lungs until the preset pressure is reached. Then, when the machine shuts off, tell the patient to remove the mouthpiece or mask and exhale completely. Repeat the process for 10 or 15 minutes each session, as ordered.

After treatment, the patient may have episodes of coughing. Assure him that coughing is both normal and beneficial.

Whenever giving IPPB therapy, stay alert for these danger signs:
• sudden drop in blood pressure accompanied by increased heart rate, possibly indicating decreased venous return to heart
• nausea
• tremors or dizziness
• rapid, shallow respirations, possibly indicating respiratory alkalosis
• distended abdomen caused by gastric insufflation
• thickening of secretions caused by inadequate humidification
• decreased respiratory rate, possibly indicating loss of hypoxic drive.

For full details on giving IPPB therapy, read the NURSING PHOTOBOOK *Providing Respiratory Care.*

---

COMPLICATIONS

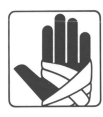

### Coping with oxygen therapy complications

You've probably administered oxygen many times to relieve hypoxia. But never consider the procedure so routine that you forget oxygen's a potent—and potentially dangerous—drug.

Oxygen therapy is too complex for us to explain in detail here. But this chart will help you quickly review its dangers. For further information, read the NURSING PHOTOBOOK *Providing Respiratory Care.*

**Complication**
Respiratory depression

**Signs and symptoms**
• Slow respiration rate

**Causes**
• Giving too high a concentration of oxygen to a patient with chronic obstructive pulmonary disease (COPD)

**Nursing considerations**
• Monitor the patient's blood gases.
• Give oxygen in low concentrations.

**Complication**
Circulatory depression

**Signs and symptoms**
• Decreased blood pressure
• Increased heart rate
• Pallor
• Cyanosis

**Causes**
• Giving oxygen until vasodilation results

**Nursing considerations**
• Monitor the patient's blood pressure.
• Check patient's central venous pressure (CVP) frequently.

**Complication**
Atelectasis

**Signs and symptoms**
• Shortness of breath
• Shallow respirations

**Causes**
• Giving oxygen at a high concentration
• Hypoventilation

**Nursing considerations**
• Make sure the patient coughs and takes deep breaths every hour.
• Hyperinflate his lungs, if necessary.

**Complication**
Oxygen toxicity

**Signs and symptoms**
• Coughing
• Pain on inspiration
• Shortness of breath
• Chest pain

**Causes**
• Giving very high oxygen concentrations with positive end expiratory pressure (PEEP) for more than 24 hours

**Nursing considerations**
• Monitor the patient's blood gases and vital signs.
• Turn patient every 2 hours.
• Improve quality of patient's ventilation with chest physiotherapy and suctioning.

## Learning about common oxygen delivery systems

Chances are, you're familiar with a variety of oxygen delivery systems: for example, the oxygen tent, the partial rebreathing mask, and the venturi mask. But the three featured here are the ones used most frequently.

Do you know their advantages and disadvantages? Can you avoid problems that may arise? Study this chart for the answers.

For more on oxygen delivery systems, see the NURSING PHOTOBOOK *Providing Respiratory Care.*

### NASAL CANNULA

**Advantages**
- Safe and simple
- Comfortable; easily tolerated
- Nasal prongs can be shaped to fit facial contour.
- Effectively delivers low oxygen concentrations
- Allows freedom of movement; doesn't interfere with eating or talking
- Inexpensive; disposable
- Can provide continuous, positive airway pressure for infants and children

**Disadvantages**
- Can't deliver oxygen concentrations greater than 40%
- Can't be used when patient has complete nasal obstructions; for example, mucosal edema or polyps
- May cause headaches or dry mucous membranes if flow rate exceeds 6 liters per minute
- Can dislodge easily
- Strap may pinch chin if adjusted too tightly.
- Patient must be alert and cooperative to help keep cannula in place.

**To avoid complications**
- Remove cannula every 8 hours, and clean it with a wet cloth. Give good mouth and nose care.
- If patient's restless, tape cannula in place.
- Check for pressure areas under nose and over ears. Apply gauze padding, if necessary.
- Moisten lips and nose with lubricating jelly, but take care not to occlude cannula.

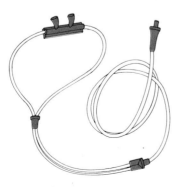

### NASAL CATHETER

**Advantages**
- Allows freedom of movement; doesn't interfere with eating or talking
- Provides stable delivery if patient's restless
- Inexpensive; disposable

**Disadvantages**
- Can't deliver oxygen concentrations greater than 45%
- May cause headaches or sinus pain if flow rate exceeds 6 liters per minute
- May dry nostrils and mucous membranes
- Catheter lumen may clog with secretions.
- Kinks easily
- Less comfortable than nasal cannula; tape may irritate skin.
- Patients lacking epiglottal reflexes may experience abdominal distention, especially at high-flow rates.

**To avoid complications**
- Change catheter every 8 hours, alternating nostrils; give good mouth and nose care.
- Check for skin irritation caused by tape.
- Use for short-term therapy.
- Moisten nose with lubricating jelly.
- Use with caution in comatose or debilitated patients.

### SIMPLE FACE MASK

**Advantages**
- Effectively delivers high oxygen concentrations
- Humidification can be increased by using large-bore tubing and aerosol mask.
- Doesn't dry mucous membranes of nose and mouth

**Disadvantages**
- Hot and confining; may irritate skin
- Tight seal necessary for higher oxygen concentration may cause discomfort.
- Interferes with eating and talking
- Can't deliver less than 40% oxygen
- Impractical for long-term therapy

**To avoid complications**
- Don't use on patient with chronic obstructive pulmonary disease (COPD).
- Place pads between mask and bony facial parts.
- Periodically massage face with fingertips.
- Wash and dry face every 2 hours.
- For adequate flush, maintain flow rate of 5 liters per minute.
- Don't adjust strap too tightly.
- Remove mask every 8 hours, and clean it with a wet cloth.

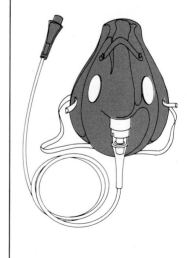

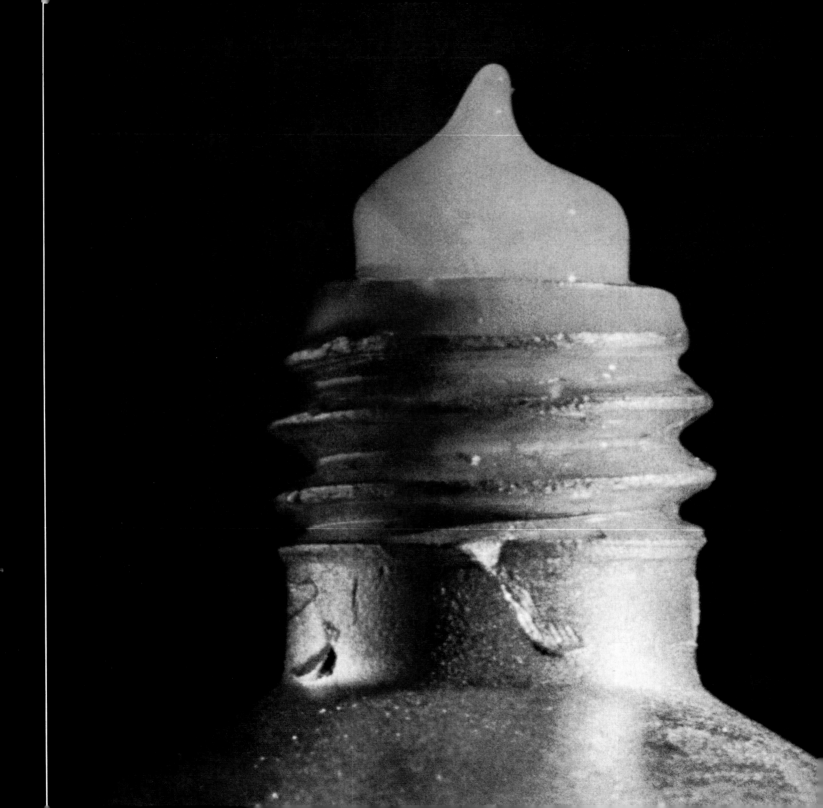

# Administering by the Dermatomucosal Route

Skin medications

Eye medications

Ear medications

Mouth and throat medications

Vaginal medications

# Dermatomucosal medications

At a time when chemo-therapeutic drugs and an-tibiotics command the medical spotlight, derma-tomucosal medications and their effects often fade in importance. But dermatomucosal medica-tions, administered prop-erly, play as vital a role in the patient's care plan as any other drugs.

Ironically, some of modern medicine's newer therapies have increased the need for effective der-matomucosal medications. Consider, for example, the patient who receives extensive antibiotic therapy. He may develop a superinfection from the antibiotics that will, in turn, require treatment with dermatomucosal medications.

Dermatomucosal medi-cations (with the excep-tion of nitroglycerin) are given for their local, not systemic, effects. Their absorption through the skin is minimal and gen-erally unpredictable.

How well a dermatomu-cosal drug is absorbed depends on the vascular-ity of the patient's skin and its thickness. Study these illustrations. As you'd expect, drug ab-sorption is greatest in skin areas with a thin epider-mal layer and many blood vessels. Drug absorption is poorest in areas with a thick epidermal layer and few blood vessels.

**Skin layers**

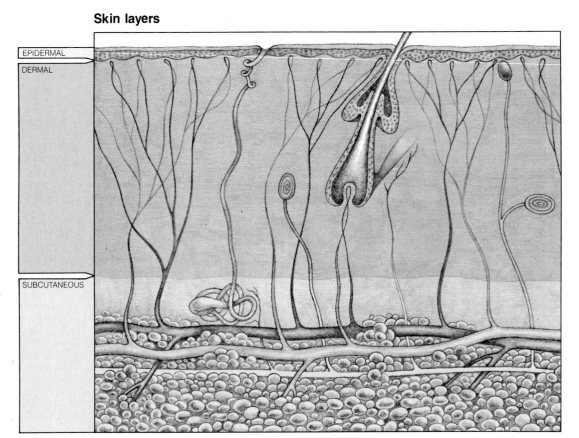

EPIDERMAL
DERMAL
SUBCUTANEOUS

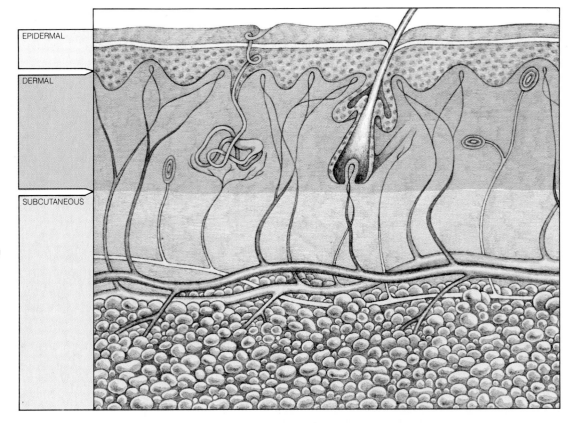

EPIDERMAL
DERMAL
SUBCUTANEOUS

# Skin medications

Applying medication to a patient's skin sounds simple. But it's really more complicated than you think. Do you know:
• how applying medication to the scalp differs from applying medication to the torso?
• why you shouldn't apply some powders and liquids to the face?
• what special precautions you must take in applying nitroglycerin ointment?
• which type of dressing to use for psoriasis?

You'll find the answers to these and many other questions you may have in this section. Study it carefully.

## Topical medications: Pros and cons

**Benefits**

• Faster relief from surface pain and itching than with systemic drugs
• Less severe allergic reactions than with systemic drugs
• Fewer side effects than with systemic drugs
• Comforting for the patient, since he can witness the care
• Increased protection against infection for skin that's lost its natural protection capabilities

**Drawbacks**

• Difficult to deliver in precise doses
• May stain skin, clothing, furniture, or bed linen
• Application procedure is time-consuming.
• May be embarrassing to patient, depending on the site
• May be difficult for the patient to apply, depending on the site

## Nurses' guide to topical dosage forms

Do you know why the doctor orders one topical dosage form over another for your patient? This chart will tell you how these dosage forms differ and how these differences affect your nursing care.

| Type | Use | Nursing considerations |
|---|---|---|
| **Powder** (an inert chemical that may contain medication) | • Promotes skin drying<br>• Reduces moisture, maceration, friction | • Apply to clean, dry skin.<br>• To prevent inhalation of powder particles, instruct patient to turn his head to one side during application.<br>• If you're applying powder to the patient's face or neck, give him a cloth or gauze to cover his mouth. Then, ask him to exhale as you apply powder. |
| **Lotion** (a suspension of insoluble powder in water or an emulsion without powder) | • Creates sensation of dryness<br>• Leaves uniform surface film of powder<br>• Soothes, cools, protects the skin | • Shake container well before using.<br>• Remove residue from previous applications, if ordered.<br>• To increase absorption in certain skin conditions, warm the patient's skin with heat packs or a bath before applying.<br>• Apply medication to clean, dry skin.<br>• Thoroughly massage lotion into the skin.<br>• After application, observe the patient's skin for local irritation. |
| **Cream** (an oil-in-water emulsion in semisolid form) | • Lubricates as a barrier | • Remove residue from previous applications, if ordered.<br>• Apply medication to clean, dry skin.<br>• Thoroughly massage cream into the skin.<br>• After application, observe the patient's skin for local irritation. |
| **Ointment** (a suspension of oil and water in semisolid form) | • Retains body heat<br>• Provides prolonged medication contact | • Remove residue from previous applications, if ordered.<br>• To increase absorption of medication, warm patient's skin with heat packs or a bath before applying.<br>• Apply medication to clean, dry skin.<br>• Apply thin layer of ointment to patient's skin, and rub it in well.<br>• Use care when applying ointment to draining wounds. |
| **Paste** (a stiff mixture of powder and ointment) | • Provides a uniform coat<br>• Reduces and repels moisture | • Remove residue from previous applications, if ordered.<br>• Apply medication to clean, dry skin.<br>• Cover medication to increase absorption and to protect the patient's clothing and bed linen. |

# Skin medications

## Unsightly skin conditions: What's your reaction?

Does your patient have an unsightly skin condition? Your reaction to it can affect the way he feels, as well as his progress toward recovery. For example, do you avoid looking at your patient or touching him? You're probably contributing to his discomfort without even realizing it.

Examine your feelings carefully. Does the thought of caring for a patient with an unsightly skin condition repel you? Accept your feelings as normal. *However, do your best not to show these feelings to your patient.* Here are some tips to help you:
• Look directly at your patient when you talk to him. Keep in mind that he probably feels more uncomfortable about his appearance than you do.
• Don't appear hesitant when you reach out to touch his affected areas during treatment. A perceptive patient will quickly sense the difference between gentleness and squeamishness.
• Don't wear gloves unless it's really necessary. Gloves may make your patient feel unclean and may hinder your ability to assess his skin condition. Before you decide if gloves are needed, ask yourself these questions: Is the patient's condition contagious? Am I allergic to the medication? Will gloves protect the patient from other infections in the unit?
• If you do wear gloves (for whatever reason), tell your patient why. *But choose your words carefully.* Don't say: "I'm wearing these gloves because you're contagious." Instead, say: "I'm wearing gloves to protect you from any germs *I may have* on my hands."

*A good rule to remember is this:* Consider how you'd feel if you were the patient with the unsightly skin condition. Then, treat your patient accordingly.

## Applying scalp medication

**1** *You're caring for a patient with psoriasis. The doctor orders triamcinolone acetonide lotion (Kenalog\*) to be applied to his scalp. Do you know how?*

First, prepare to wash the patient's hair and scalp with a mild shampoo. If he's on bed rest, place a waterproof drape underneath his head and a washbasin by his bed.

Then, thoroughly shampoo his hair and scalp, using only your fingertips to massage his scalp. Don't use your fingernails, even if you're wearing gloves. Doing so could worsen his condition.

Rinse, and repeat the procedure.

*Note:* If your patient can shampoo his own hair and scalp, let him. But be sure to instruct him to lather twice and rinse thoroughly.

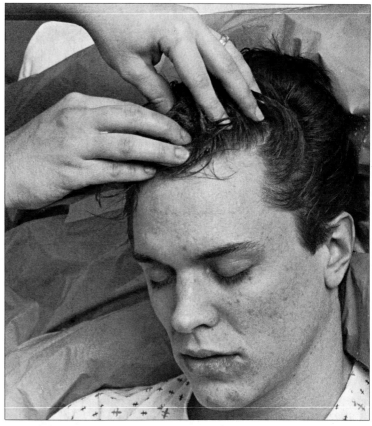

**2** Carefully dry his hair and scalp with a towel. Comb his hair to eliminate any tangles.

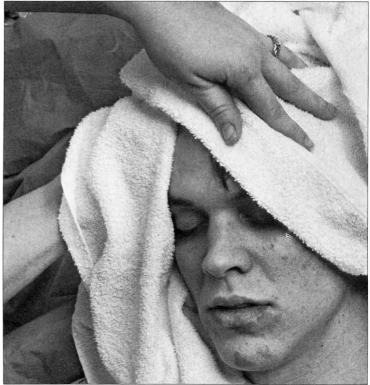

*Available in the United States and in Canada.

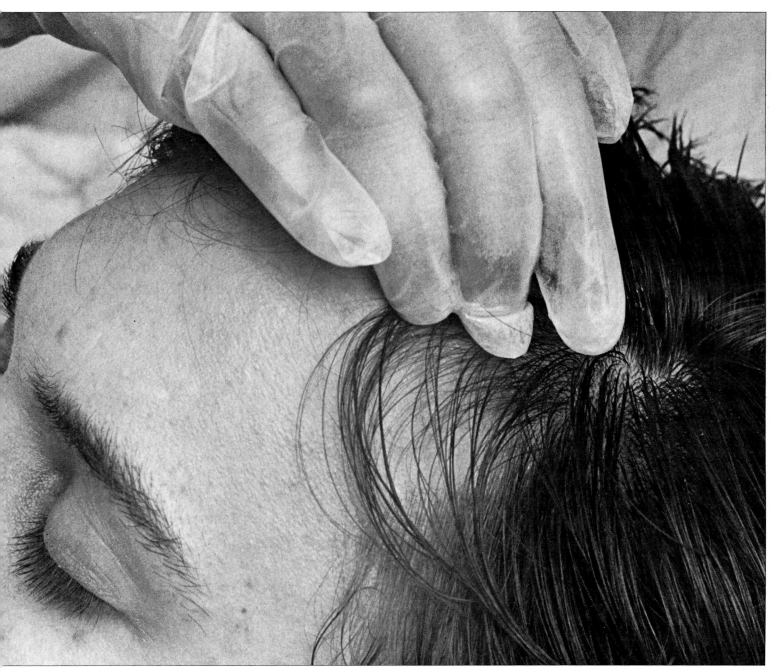

**3** Now you're ready to apply the medication. Put on a pair of gloves, if you haven't already. Use a comb to part your patient's hair naturally. Then, apply a liberal amount of medication to your fingertips, and spread it evenly on his exposed scalp. Part his hair again, about ½" (1.3 cm) from the original part. Repeat the application. Continue this procedure until you've applied medication to his entire scalp. Massage the medication into his scalp, unless ordered otherwise.

Repeat the shampoo procedure, if the instructions on the medication label call for it. Rinse the patient's hair and scalp thoroughly. Finally, document the entire procedure, as well as your observations, in your nurses' notes.

# Skin medications

### Applying facial medication

**1** *The doctor admits Helen Daniels to treat her uncontrolled hypertension. During her hospitalization, he determines that she's also suffering from eczematous dermatitis. To treat this condition, the doctor wants you to apply betamethasone valerate (Valisone\*) to Mrs. Daniels' face. Do you know how?*

First, check the medication to make sure it matches the order. Then, explain the procedure to the patient.

Position the patient so she's comfortable, and provide her with as much privacy as possible. If you plan to wear gloves, use snug-fitting surgical gloves rather than loose, plastic protective ones. The snug fit will make it easier to apply the medication.

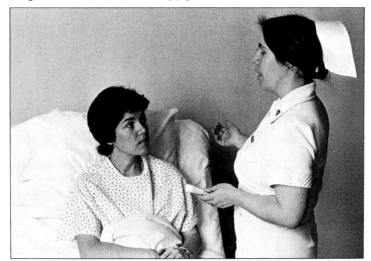

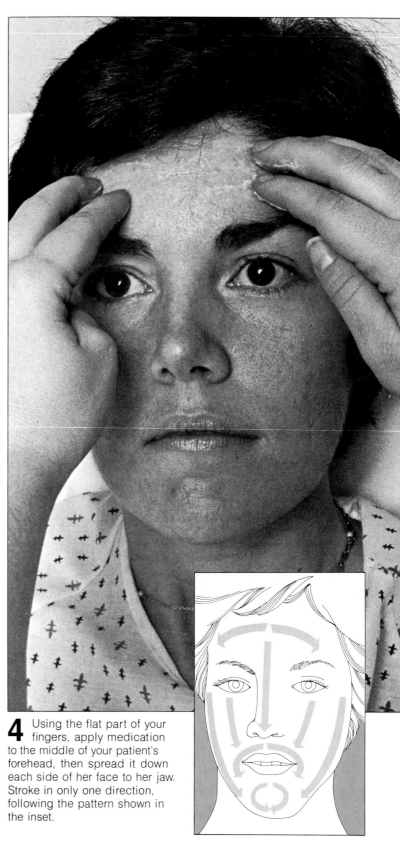

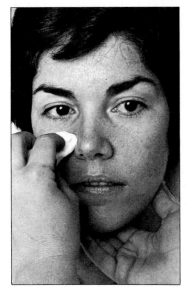

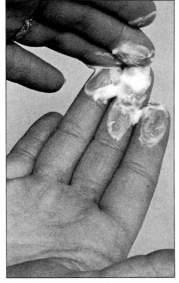

**2** Examine the patient's skin. Is it clean of previous medication or dried exudate? If not, gently wash her face with mild soap and water. Or gently massage it with normal saline solution, peroxide, cottonseed oil, or mineral oil.

**3** When the skin's prepared, open the medication container. Rub a small amount of medication over the inner aspects of your fingers.

**4** Using the flat part of your fingers, apply medication to the middle of your patient's forehead, then spread it down each side of her face to her jaw. Stroke in only one direction, following the pattern shown in the inset.

\*Available in the United States and in Canada.

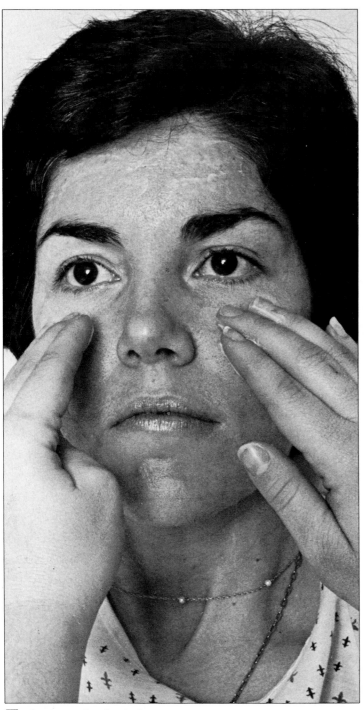

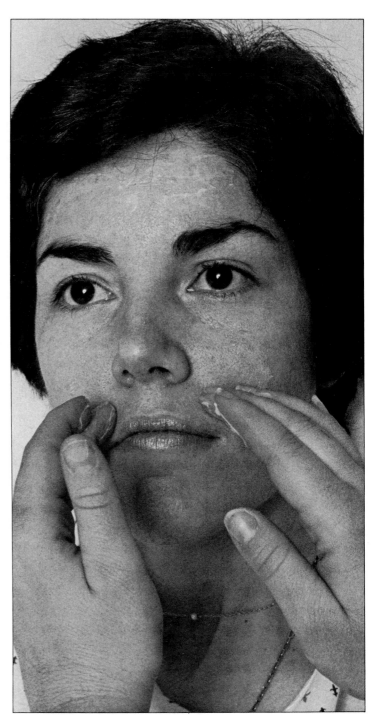

**5** Apply medication below the patient's eyes, working down her cheeks to her chin. *Important:* Never let the medication come in contact with the eyes. To avoid this risk, doctors rarely order thin solutions or emulsions for the face.

**6** Using a very small amount, apply the medication under the patient's nose, around her mouth (avoiding the lips), and over her chin. Don't rub.

Finally, cap the medication. Document the entire procedure, along with your observations, in your nurses' notes.

# Skin medications

### Applying body medication

**1** *You're caring for a patient with dermatitis. To treat your patient's condition, the doctor has ordered betamethasone benzoate (Benisone), a medicated body cream. Do you know how to apply the medication? Follow the same procedure we outlined for applying medication to the face (see pages 124 and 125). Only the spreading technique differs.*

Begin the procedure by checking the medication against the order. Then, tell the patient what you're going to do and why.

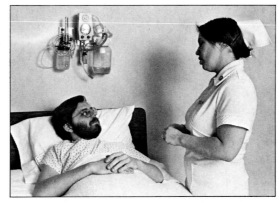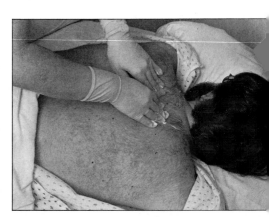

**2** Place the patient in a comfortable position. Draw a curtain around his bed to assure privacy. Protect the bed linen with bedsaver pads.

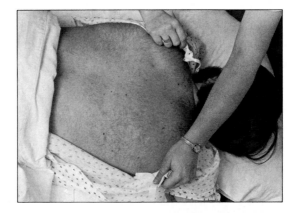

**3** Next, examine his skin for dried exudate or residue from previous medication applications. If you find any, remove it with mild soap and water, or use a sterile gauze pad soaked in normal saline solution or mineral oil.

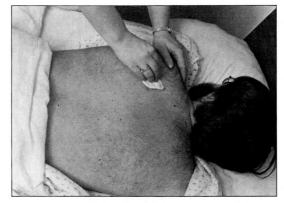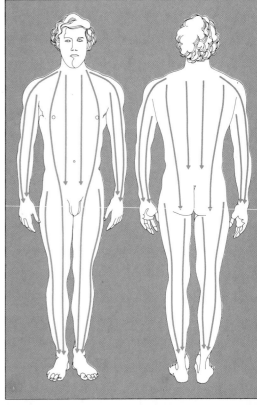

**4** Put on a pair of sterile gloves, and remove a generous amount of medication from its container. Warm the medication by rubbing it between your fingers.

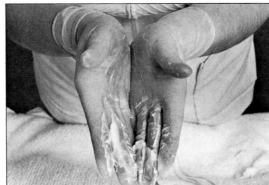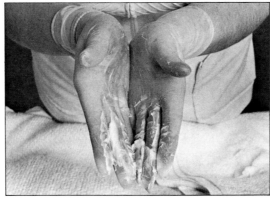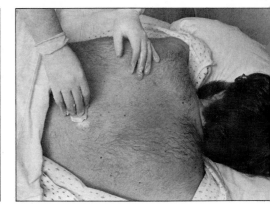

**5** Begin applying the medication at the midline of the patient's neck. Spread it laterally down his back, toward his buttocks, as shown in this photo. This method follows normal hair growth patterns and minimizes the tingling sensation that occurs when creams and ointments are applied with random strokes.

**6** Follow the application pattern shown here if you're applying medication to the patient's chest, arms, or legs.

**7** Use a clean gauze pad and downward strokes to remove any excess cream, especially in areas where it can collect; for example, under a female patient's breasts, or in between skin rolls of obese patients. Finally, document the procedure. And, remember: change the bed linen as necessary.

*Note:* Is your patient undergoing long-term treatment with a steroid ointment? He may experience unintended systemic effects from the medication; for example, adrenal insufficiency. Notify the doctor if your patient shows any of these signs: anorexia, weakness, nausea, or vomiting.

## Applying nitroglycerin ointment

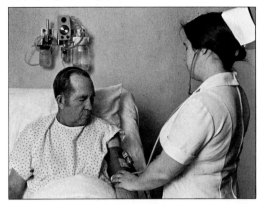

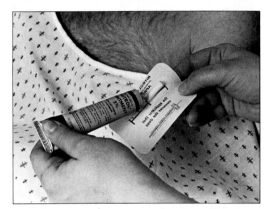

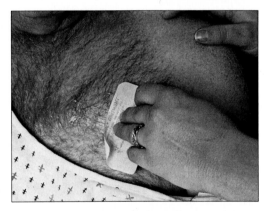

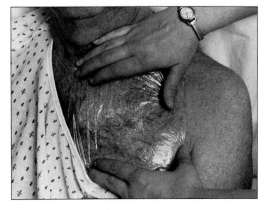

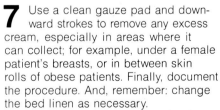

**1** *Unlike other medications applied to the skin, nitroglycerin ointment is used for its systemic, not local, effect. You'll use nitroglycerin ointment to dilate the veins and arteries of a patient with cardiac ischemia or angina pectoris in order to increase the blood flow to his heart. Here's how to apply nitroglycerin ointment:*

Take a reading of your patient's blood pressure, so you have it to compare with later readings.

**2** Next, gather your equipment. Nitroglycerin ointment, which is prescribed in inches, comes with a rectangular piece of ruled paper, to be used in applying the medication. Confirm the medication order by checking it against the patient's Kardex. Then, squeeze the prescribed amount of ointment onto the ruled paper, as shown here.

*Note:* As an added precaution, you may want to wear gloves to avoid coming in contact with the medication and absorbing it systemically.

**3** Use the paper to apply the medication to the patient's skin (usually on his chest or arm). Spread a thin layer of the ointment over a 3" (7.6 cm) area.

**4** For increased absorption, cover the site with plastic wrap.

After 5 minutes, take the patient's blood pressure. If it's dropped significantly, and your patient has a headache (from vasodilation of blood vessels in his head), notify the doctor immediately. He'll probably want to decrease the next dose.

If the patient's blood pressure has dropped (but he shows no side effects), instruct him to lie still until it returns to normal.

Finally, document the procedure and your observations in your nurses' notes.

# Skin medications

### Applying a debriding agent

**1** *You'll apply a debriding agent to a patient's wound, burn, or decubitus ulcer to dissolve purulent or necrotic tissue. Agents commonly prescribed for this purpose are dextranomer (Debrisan), which is made up of granular particles and applied to a wound or an ulcer; and fibrinolysin and desoxyribonuclease (Elase\*), which is an ointment used on encrusted lesions.*

Suppose you're using dextranomer to treat a decubitus ulcer. Assemble this equipment: dextranomer, glycerin ointment, gloves, a tongue depressor, normal saline solution, hydrogen peroxide, a bedsaver pad, several 4" x 4" sterile gauze pads, and a roll of gauze. Put on the gloves, and remove the dressing from the ulcer.

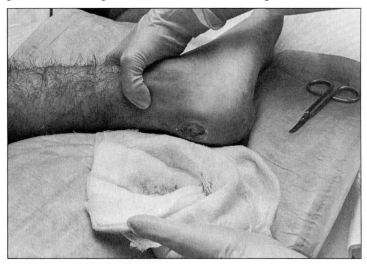

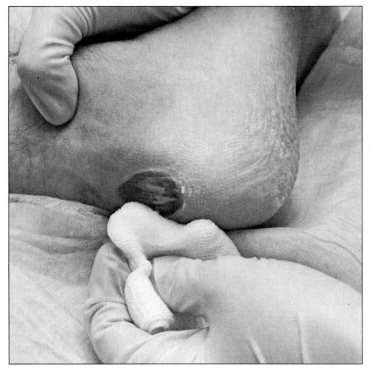

**2** Flush the ulcer with normal saline solution, then hydrogen peroxide, to remove loose debris and previously applied medication. Let the ulcer remain wet.

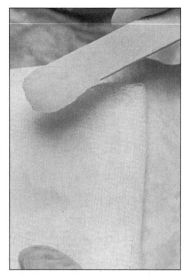

**3** Now, place the dextranomer in the center of a sterile gauze pad, add some glycerin ointment, and mix the two with a tongue depressor. This makes a paste that will adhere well to the ulcer.

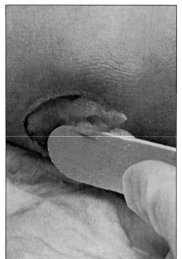

**4** Use the tongue depressor to apply the paste evenly to the ulcer. Take care not to get paste on healthy tissue. As a precaution, wipe excess paste from the site with a gauze pad. Then, apply petroleum jelly to the healthy skin to protect it.

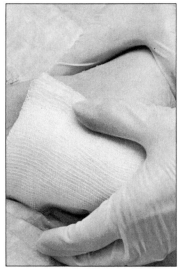

**5** Cover the ulcer with a fresh sterile gauze pad, and secure it with gauze. Don't wrap the gauze too tightly, because the dextranomer paste will expand.

*Important:* Never tape the gauze pad, because the tape could further irritate the patient's already tender skin.

Repeat the entire procedure at least once a day—but preferably two or three times daily—until the ulcer is debrided. Changing the dressing hastens the debriding process, because necrotic tissue is removed with the gauze pad.

\*Available in the United States and in Canada.

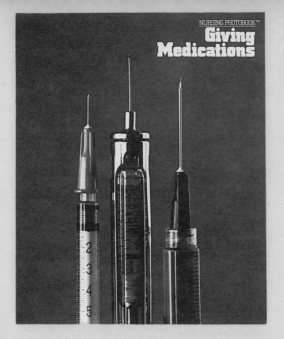

**NURSING PHOTOBOOK™**
**Giving Medications**

## Use this card to subscribe to the NURSING PHOTOBOOK™ series.

☐ **YES.** I want to subscribe to the series and save $2.00 on each book I buy. Please send me *Giving Medications* as my first volume. If I decide to keep it, I will pay $13.95 plus shipping and handling. I understand that I will receive an exciting new Photobook approximately every other month on the same 10-day, free-examination basis. Each volume I decide to keep costs just $13.95 (plus shipping and handling). There is no minimum number of books I must buy, and I may cancel my subscription at any time.

If I choose not to keep *Giving Medications,* I will return it within 10 days and owe nothing.

Name _____

Address _____

City _____

State or
Province _____    Zip or
Mail Code _____

---

## 10-DAY FREE TRIAL

## USE THESE CARDS TO:

1. **Join the NURSING PHOTOBOOK™ series, with *Giving Medications* as your first volume. $13.95 per book.**

   *or*

2. **Buy extra copies of *Giving Medications* without joining the series. $15.95 per book.**

## Use this card to buy *Giving Medications* without joining the series.

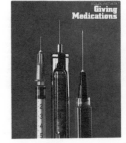

Please send me *Giving Medications* to examine for 10 days free. If I keep the book, I pay $15.95, plus shipping and handling. If I do not keep the book, I will return it within 10 days and owe nothing. Please send me _____ copies and bill me.

Name _____

Address _____

City _____

State or
Province _____    Zip or
Mail Code _____

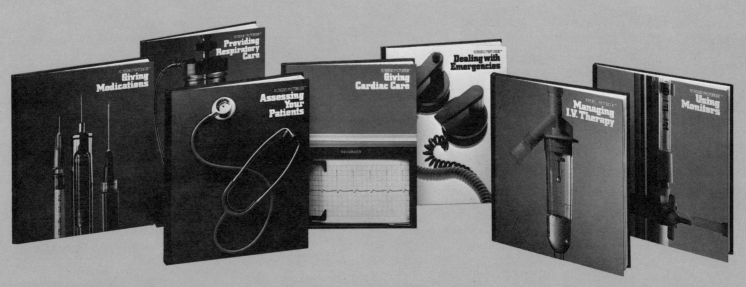

**Each Photobook shows you step-by-step how to carry out important nursing procedures.**

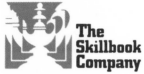
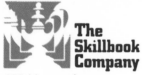
*Giving Medications...your* **introduction to the brand-new NURSING PHOTOBOOK™ series.**

...the remarkable breakthrough in nursing education that can change your career. Each book in this unique series contains detailed *Photostories...* and tables, charts, and graphs to help you learn important new procedures. And each handsome Photobook offers you • 160 illustrated, fact-filled pages • brilliant, high-contrast photographs • convenient 9″ × 10½″ size • durable, hardcover binding • carefully chosen bibliography • complete index. Watch the experts at work showing you how to... administer drugs... teach your patient about his illness and its treatment... minimize trauma... understand doctors' diagnoses... increase patient comfort... and much more. Discover how you can become a better nurse by joining this exciting series.

## 10-DAY FREE TRIAL

## USE THESE CARDS TO:

1. **Join the NURSING PHOTOBOOK™ series, with *Giving Medications* as your first volume. $13.95 per book.**

*or*

2. **Buy extra copies of *Giving Medications* without joining the series. $15.95 per book.**

## Here's what nurses are saying about this exciting new series:

"The step-by-step approach makes everything clear. It's the best 'how-to' guide to nursing on the market today."
—RN, Tex.

"On night duty, there are very few people to help me set up equipment. That's when I really depend on this series."
—RN, Wyo.

"I'm learning more from each Photobook than I learned in nursing school."
—RN, Utah

"Marvelous idea! It's better than a demonstration because it lets me study each procedure as long as I wish."
—RN, La.

"Your photos and illustrations make me feel like I'm the one doing the procedures."
—RN, Calif.

"The nursing tips are indispensable. They make the difference between good and expert care."
—RN, Mich.

### GUARANTEE OF SATISFACTION

Each volume in this series is guaranteed by *Nursing81*—thoroughly and without reservations. You have the right to examine each volume for 10 days. Try the various procedures shown. Show the book to others for their opinions. Use the book as a tool to improve your everyday work, if you wish. We believe so strongly that it will show you new and better ways to practice nursing that we're extending this no-risk opportunity to every subscriber.

If you don't find any book helpful, simply return it within 10 days. You'll owe nothing. We thereby guarantee that you'll be satisfied with what you accept... or you won't owe a cent.

# Patient teaching

# Home care

## How to apply a medicated cream or ointment

Dear Patient:

To help treat your _____
condition, your doctor wants you to apply

_____
cream/ointment to your _____
The nurse has shown you the proper way to apply it. When you apply the medication yourself, follow the directions on the label, and observe these guidelines:

• Wash your hands thoroughly before beginning the procedure.

• Use warm water and soap to cleanse the skin of any old cream/ointment.

• When you uncap the container, place the cap so the grooved side is up.

• Apply the cream/ointment as directed.

• Do/don't cover the area with a loose/tight dressing.

• Notify the doctor if you notice any of the following: a change in the amount, color, consistency, or odor of drainage; or increased swelling or redness.

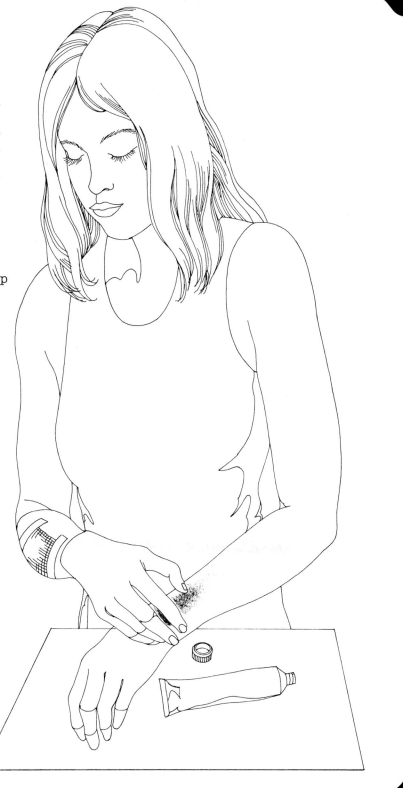

# Skin medications

## Nurses' guide to medicated baths

What if your patient suffers from widespread itching and you want to give him relief? Consider getting an order for a medicated tub bath. It's the most effective way to treat large body surfaces quickly. It can also:
• provide immersion to remove debris, exudate, and necrotic tissue.
• hydrate the wound.
• soften scales and crust to ease removal.
• leave a thin film of medication on the patient's skin.
• cleanse and treat tender skin gently, without the friction of a sponge bath.

The medicated tub bath's only drawback is its inconvenience. A bath takes time to prepare and administer.

Begin by making sure the tub room is warm, private, and draft-free. Make sure the tub has been cleaned and disinfected. Explain the procedure to the patient.

Next, fill the tub about two-thirds full with warm water (about 15 gallons [57 liters]). Check the temperature to make sure it's 100° to 105° F. (37.8° to 40.6° C.). Using the chart below as a guide, add the medication ordered by the doctor.

| Type | Example | Mix | Purpose | Procedure |
|---|---|---|---|---|
| Colloidal preparation | Oatmeal (Aveeno Colloidal) | 1 cup (226.8 g) in 15 gallons | Antipruritic | Mix the oatmeal with small amounts of cool water to form a paste. Gradually, add the paste to the water as the tub is filling. |
| Starch preparation | Cornstarch | 1 cup (226.8 g) in 15 gallons | Antipruritic | Slowly dissolve the powder in a small amount of water, then add it to the tub. |
| Soda preparation | Baking soda | ½ cup (113.4 g) in 15 gallons | Antipruritic | Stir the powder into standing water until it's dissolved. |
| Oil preparation | Cottonseed oil | 2 oz (59 ml) in 15 gallons | Relieves itching from dry skin | Stir the liquid into standing water until it's suspended. |
| Tablet | Potassium permanganate | 5 g in 15 gallons | Deodorizer | Dissolve tablets in small amount of water to make a solution. Stir the solution into standing water. *Note:* May stain the patient's skin. Remove stain with a dilute acid, such as lemon juice. |

After you've added the medication, disperse it throughout the tub water. Check the water temperature again to make sure it's correct. Help your patient into the tub, and bathe him for about 20 minutes. Then, assist him out of the tub, taking care that he doesn't slip from the film left on the tub by the medication. Use a clean towel to pat the excess medication from his body. Guard your patient against chilling. Remember, the patient with a skin condition loses body heat rapidly. Finally, clean and disinfect the tub, so it's ready for the next patient.

The doctor may want the patient to continue medicated bath treatments at home. If he does, make sure the patient understands the procedure.

Suppose the doctor's ordered a warm-water sitz bath for your patient. Teach him how to use one by following the procedure that's outlined on the opposite page. Then, copy and complete the home care aid so he can take it home.

## Selecting the right dressing

You'll use a medicated dressing to treat a patient's skin problems for one or more of the following reasons: when he can't tolerate a bath; when the condition's in an area that can't be soaked; or when the condition needs long-term treatment and protection.

Study this chart to learn about the different types of dressings you can use. Be sure to apply the dressing correctly. Incorrect application can macerate the site and stain clothing and linen.

| Type | Description | Used for | Medicinal effects or benefits |
|---|---|---|---|
| Open, wet dressing (unoccluded) | A dressing soaked in medication, applied to the skin, and left uncovered. When the water in the medication evaporates, the dressing is remoistened. Used, for example, to apply a solution of water and aluminum sulfate (Domeboro Powder*). | • Acute inflammatory skin conditions, erosions, ulcers<br>• Skin lesions, with oozing exudate | • Delivers medication<br>• Softens and heals the skin<br>• Soaks up pus and exudate<br>• Decreases blood flow to inflamed areas<br>• Helps promote drainage<br>• Protects site from contamination |
| Closed, wet dressing (occluded) | A dressing soaked in medication, applied to the skin, and covered with either an occlusive or insulative bandage. By covering the dressing this way, you prevent water evaporation and heat loss. The occlusive dressing is used to apply desoximetasone (Topicort*). The insulative dressing is used to apply boric acid solution. | • Cellulitis<br>• Erysipelas<br>• Psoriasis<br>• Lichen simplex chronicus<br>• Eczema | • Delivers medication<br>• Softens and heals the skin<br>• Increases effectiveness of medication<br>• Soaks up pus and exudate<br>• Increases blood flow to inflamed areas<br>• Protects site from contamination |
| Wet to dry dressing | Same as open, wet dressing, except the dressing is removed after water evaporation, not remoistened. Used, for example, to apply sodium hypochlorite (Dakin's solution). | • Wound irrigation | • Delivers medication<br>• Softens the skin<br>• Soaks up pus, exudate, debris, eschar<br>• Protects site from contamination |
| Dry dressing | An ordinary gauze pad applied to the skin. Used, for example, with debriding agent, collagenase (Collagenase ABC). | • Neurodermatitis<br>• Stasis dermatitis | • Protects skin from abrasion<br>• Protects site from contamination |

*Available in the United States and in Canada.

# Patient teaching

# Home care

## Giving yourself a sitz bath

**1** Dear Patient:
When you go home, the doctor wants you to take warm-water sitz baths to soothe your rectal irritation. Take a sitz bath at these times: _____

_____

If the doctor orders, add this medication to the warm water:

_____

For your convenience, we've provided you with a sitz bath kit. It contains a plastic pan and a plastic bag with attached tubing. Here's how to use it:

First, raise the toilet seat, and fit the plastic pan onto the toilet bowl. Position the pan so its drainage holes are along the back of the bowl, as shown here. If you've placed the pan correctly, you'll see a single slot in front.

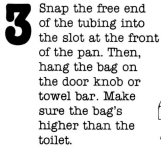

**3** Snap the free end of the tubing into the slot at the front of the pan. Then, hang the bag on the door knob or towel bar. Make sure the bag's higher than the toilet.

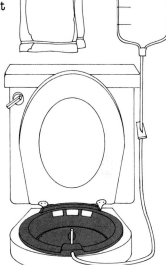

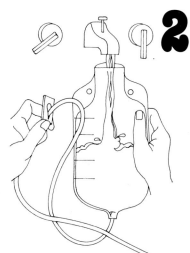

**2** Next, close the clamp on the bag's tubing. Fill the bag with warm water and medication (if ordered).

**4** Now, you're ready for your sitz bath. Sit in the pan, and open the clamp on the tubing. Let the warm water flow from the bag and fill the pan. (Don't worry about it overflowing, because excess water will flow out the drainage holes.) Continue to sit in the pan until the water begins to cool. After your sitz bath, dry yourself completely. If ordered by the doctor, apply an ointment or dressing.

# Eye medications

Basically, administering eye medications involves simple procedures. But the technical details require your special attention. For example, when you're instilling eye drops, do you know which part of the eye to use? Where should you instill eye ointment? What side effects may your patient experience?

These questions and many others are answered on the following pages. While you're reading this section, keep these tips in mind:
• Always use clean technique, because an eyedropper is easily contaminated.
• Always warm eye solutions to room temperature before administering.
• Be especially careful not to injure the patient's cornea during the procedure.

If you'd like to learn more, read on.

## How to perform eye irrigation

**1** *The doctor may want you to irrigate your patient's eye for one of three reasons: to treat inflammation or infection, to flush away contaminants or foreign bodies, or to prepare the patient for surgery. This photostory will show you how.*

After washing your hands, gather the necessary equipment. You'll need a plastic irrigation syringe and bulb, an emesis basin, rayon balls or 4" x 4" sterile gauze pads, a towel, and a bedsaver pad. In addition, you'll need the prescribed ophthalmic solution, which is usually an isotonic solution like normal saline or lactated Ringer's. Whatever medication you're using, make sure it's sterile and not outdated. Then, warm the solution to room temperature.

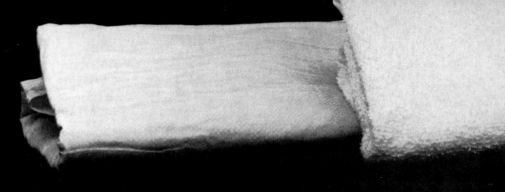

**2** Take time to reassure your patient and explain what you're going to do. Have her lie on her side in a comfortable position, with her affected eye closest to the bed. This way, fluid drainage won't contaminate her other eye.

Place a bedsaver pad under her head and neck, and an emesis basin and towel beside her face to catch the drainage.

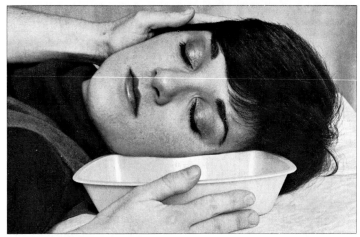

**3** Check for contact lenses. Next, moisten a gauze pad with sterile saline solution, and use it to gently clean any secretions from the patient's eyelids. When you work, always wipe from the inner to the outer canthus.

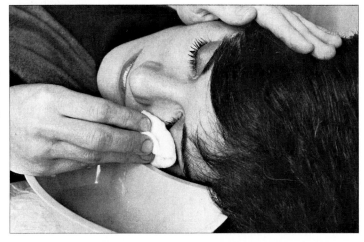

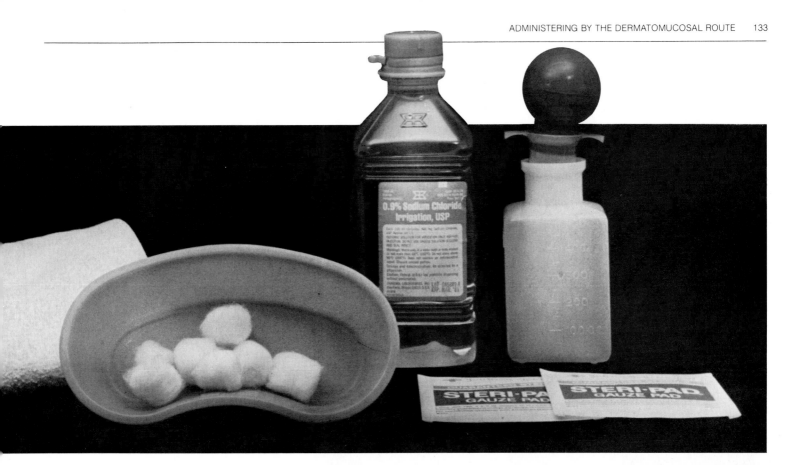

**4** Now, you're ready to begin the irrigation. Using one hand, hold the patient's eyelids open with your thumb and index finger, taking care not to press on her eyeball. With your other hand, hold the solution-filled irrigation syringe. Ask the patient to look away from the tip of the syringe. Then, squeeze the bulb to direct a stream of fluid across her eye, from the inner to the outer canthus. To prevent corneal damage and maintain sterility, avoid touching the patient's eye or eyelids with the syringe tip.

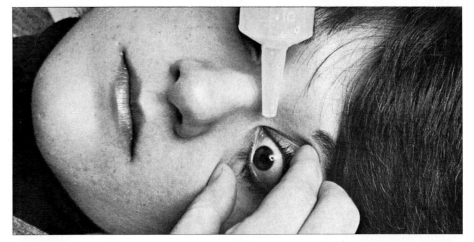

**5** When you need to use a large quantity of irrigating solution, prepare an I.V. setup at the patient's bedside. Remove the needle from an I.V. line, and attach the line to a 1,000 ml bottle of the prescribed solution. Use the flow clamp to adjust the flow rate to a gentle stream. Then, irrigate your patient's eye, as shown in this photo. Pause periodically throughout the procedure to help your patient relax.

When you've finished the irrigation, gently dry the patient's eyelids and face with the gauze pads or rayon balls. Discard the used solution. Then, document the entire procedure, as well as your observations, in your nurses' notes.

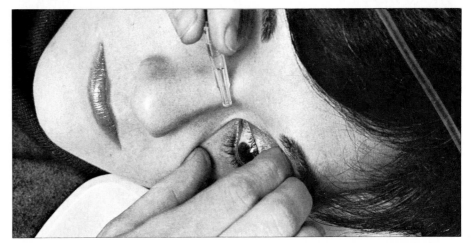

# Eye medications

## How to instill eyedrops

**1** *Your patient has glaucoma, and you've been instructed to give her two drops of pilocarpine hydrochloride\* (Pilocar) each day. Do you know how? Read this photostory.*

First, make sure you have the correct drug and that it's not outdated. Check the label to make sure it reads FOR OPHTHALMIC USE.

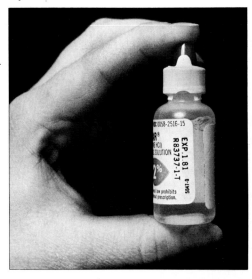

**2** Then, hold the bottle up to the light to check the solution for possible color change or sediment. If it looks peculiar, return it to the pharmacy and order a fresh bottle.

Warm the solution to room temperature just before beginning the procedure. Then, wash your hands thoroughly.

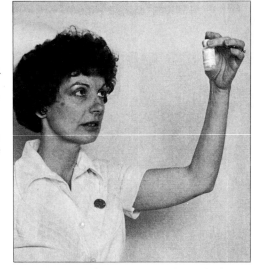

**3** Next, prepare the patient. For her comfort, have her lie on her back. Meanwhile, explain what you're going to do. Moisten a sterile gauze pad with normal saline solution, and gently clean her eyelids and lashes to remove any crust or secretions.

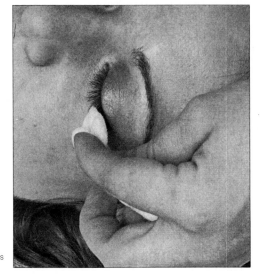

*\*Available in the United States and in Canada.*

**4** Ask the patient to tilt her head back and slightly toward the side with the affected eye. This will prevent the solution from flowing in her tear duct. Be especially careful about this if you're using a medication like atropine, because it can prove toxic if it's absorbed in the patient's system.

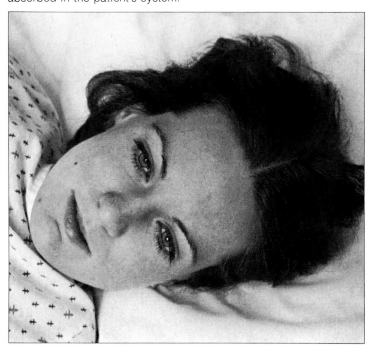

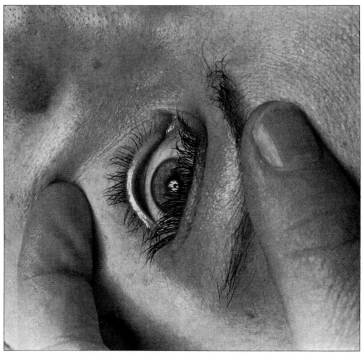

**5** Ask your patient to look up and focus on a specific object. Place your index finger on your patient's cheekbone and gently pull down her skin, exposing the lower conjunctival sac. Take care not to press on her eyeball.

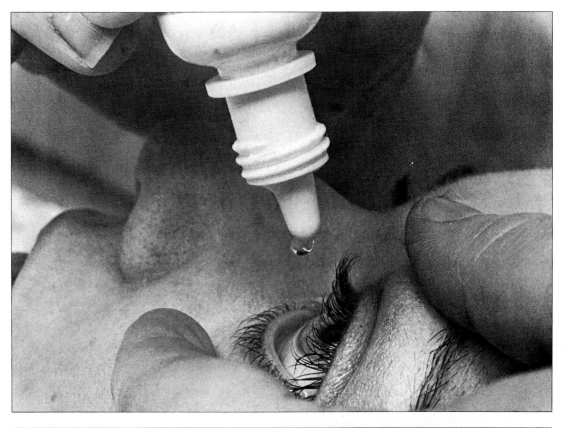

**6** Now, with your other hand, hold the eyedropper or squeeze bottle near the outer canthus of her eye. But don't let the tip touch her eyeball or eyelashes.

Squeeze the prescribed number of drops into the conjunctival sac. To prevent possible damage, never place drops directly on the patient's cornea.

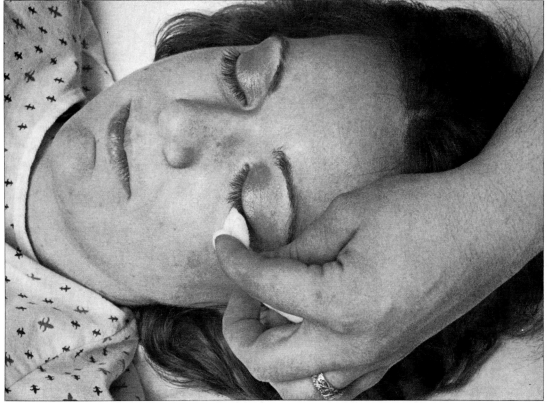

**7** Release the patient's eyelid, and let her blink to distribute the medication over her eye and inner lids. Use a rayon ball or a tissue to blot away any excess fluid, working from the inner canthus out.

Repeat the entire procedure on the other eye, if ordered. Remember, always use a fresh rayon ball or tissue to clean the other eye.

Caution your patient not to rub her eyes. Observe her closely for any side effects that may be caused by the medication.

Finally, give her a completed copy of the home care aid on the page 139. Let her administer the next dose, as you stand by to help and encourage her.

# Eye medications

### How to instill eye ointment

**1** *Let's say you're going to give eye ointment to your patient. Before you do, make sure you have the correct medication and that it's not outdated. Check the tube for the words* FOR OPHTHALMIC USE. *Why? Because ophthalmic drugs are made with a special, nonirritating base suitable for the eye's sensitive tissues.*

Warm the tube to room temperature. Now you're ready to begin the procedure.

First, wash your hands. Then, position your patient on her back. Take the time to reassure her and tell her what you're going to do. Explain that her vision will be temporarily blurred by the ointment, but that such blurring is normal and will disappear.

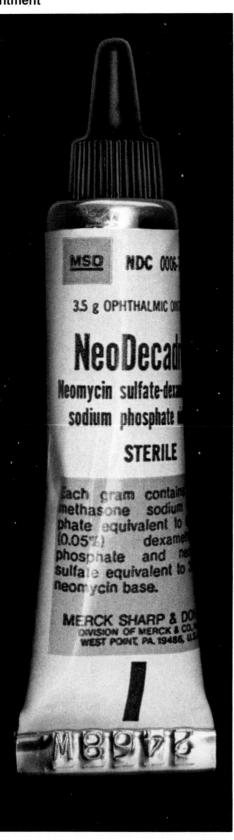

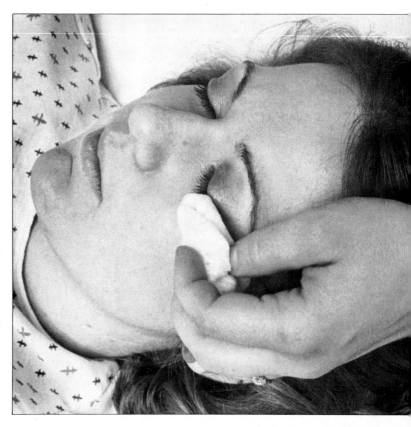

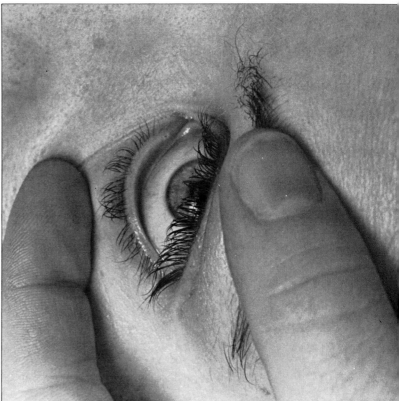

**2** Moisten a sterile gauze pad with normal saline solution. Gently clean the patient's eyelids and lashes of any crust, secretions, or old ointment. When you've finished, tilt her head back, and urge her to relax. Remove the cap from the ointment tube, taking care not to contaminate either.

**4** Now, squeeze a thin ribbon of ointment along the conjunctival sac, starting at the inner canthus. As you approach the eye's outer canthus, rotate the tube to detach the ointment.

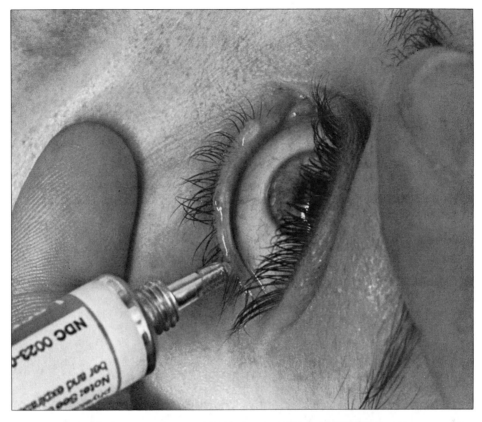

**3** Ask your patient to look up and focus on a specific object. With one hand, place your index finger on the patient's cheekbone. Gently pull down on her skin to expose the conjunctival sac.

**5** Release the patient's lower lid. Ask her to close her eyes for 1 to 2 minutes, so the medication can spread and be absorbed. Use a rayon ball or a tissue to gently wipe away any excess medication. Finally, document the procedure, including your observations, in your nurses' notes.

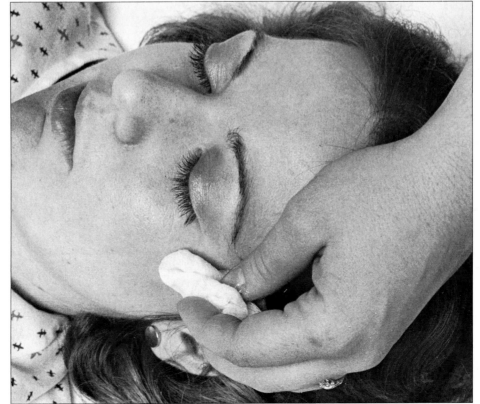

# Eye medications

## Applying an eye patch

**1** *Have you been administering ophthalmic medication to your patient? If so, the doctor may also want you to apply an eye patch. Here's how:*

First, wash your hands. Then, ask the patient to close both eyes. Use as many sterile gauze pads as you need to fill her orbital space. This will provide a base for the patch.

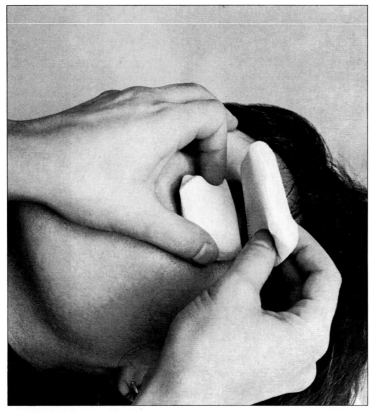

**2** Next, grasp the sterile eye patch in the center, and place it over the gauze pads. Then, apply benzoin to her cheekbone, as the nurse is doing here.

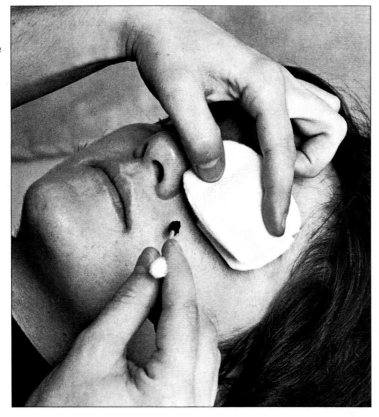

**3** Secure the patch with two parallel strips of nonallergenic tape, preferably plastic, like Dermicel®. Work from the patient's midforehead to her cheekbone, as the nurse is doing here.

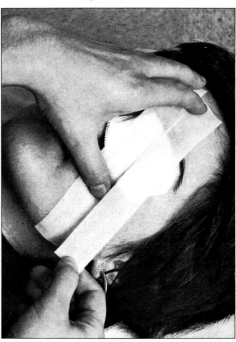

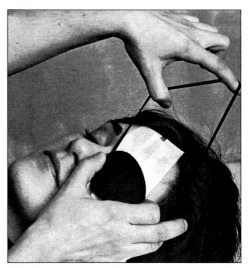

**4** Does the patient's eye require extra protection? Apply a black eye patch on top of the regular eye patch, as shown here.

When it's time to instill the next dose of medication, remove the patch by loosening the tape from the forehead down. If you notice any drainage on the gauze or the patch, document your findings on the patient's chart.

Replace the gauze pads and patch (if soiled) each time you instill medication.

# Patient teaching

## Home care

### Giving yourself eye drops

Dear Patient:

To relieve your eye infection or irritation, your doctor has prescribed these eye drops: _____

_____

Use them exactly as directed on the label. Here's how:
- Begin by washing your hands thoroughly.
- Hold the bottle up to the light and examine it. If the medication's discolored or contains sediment, discard it immediately and have the prescription refilled. If it looks OK, warm the medication to room temperature by holding the bottle between your hands for 2 minutes.
- Next, moisten a rayon ball or tissue with water, and clean all secretions from around your eyes. Use a fresh rayon ball or tissue for each eye, so you don't spread infection.
- Now, stand or sit before a mirror, or lie on your back, whichever's most comfortable for you. Squeeze the bulb of the eyedropper to fill the dropper with medication.
- Tilt your head slightly back and toward the eye you're treating. Pull down your lower eyelid. (Don't pull your upper eyelid, or you'll put unnecessary pressure on your eye.)
- Position the dropper over the conjunctival sac you've exposed between your lower lid and the white of your eye. Steady your hand by resting two fingers against your cheek or nose.
- Look away from the dropper.

Then, squeeze the prescribed number of drops into the sac. Don't drop the medication directly onto your eyeball. Take care not to touch the dropper to your eye or eyelashes. Wipe away excess medication with a clean tissue.
- Repeat the procedure in the other eye, if the doctor orders.
- Recap the medication. Store the bottle away from light and extreme heat.

Important: Call your doctor immediately if you notice any of these side effects: _____

_____

And remember, never put any medication in your eyes unless the label reads FOR OPHTHALMIC USE or FOR USE IN THE EYES.

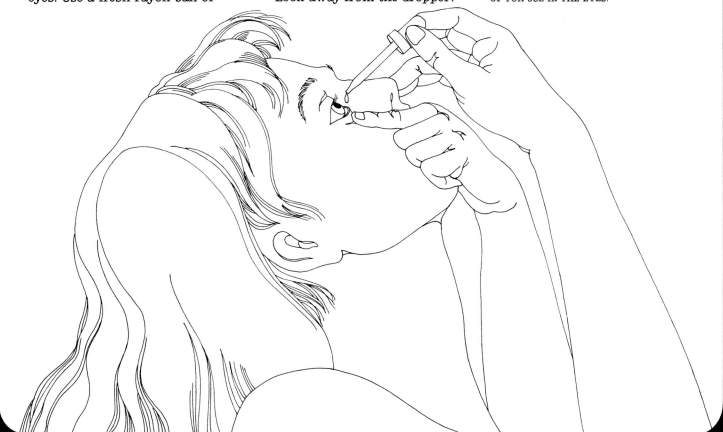

# Ear medications

Before you administer any ear medication, test your knowledge by answering these questions:
• How warm should an ear medication be before it's administered?
• What's the proper technique for straightening an ear canal? How do you adjust this technique when your patient's a child?
• Why should you direct ear drops to the side of the ear canal?
• What complication might occur if you don't clean around the ear after you irrigate it?

These questions and many more are answered in the following pages. Read on to find out about giving ear medications.

## How to irrigate the ear

**1** *Suppose your patient has wax impacted in her ear and has been using triethanolamine polypeptide oleate-condensate (Cerumenex*) to soften it. After the softening process has had time to take place, you'll instill a solution of hydrogen peroxide and water (or warm water only) to clean out the wax. Here's how:*

Seat the patient upright. Tilt her head slightly to one side to expose the affected ear. Drape towels over her shoulder and around her neck. Instruct her to hold an emesis basin under her ear.

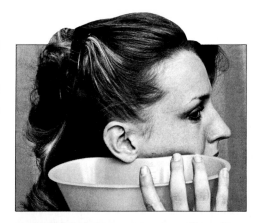

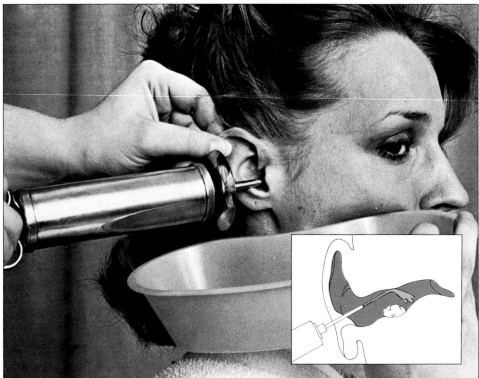

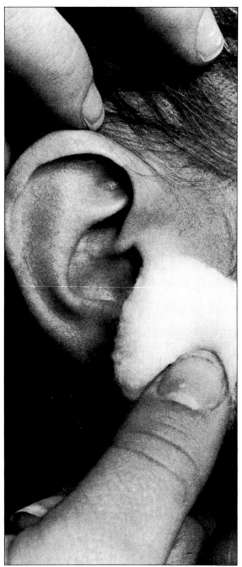

**2** Pull the auricle *up and back* to straighten the canal. With an ear syringe, instill approximately 50 ml warmed solution into the patient's ear. Direct the stream toward the *top* of the ear canal, not toward the tympanic membrane, as shown in the inset. Don't exert too much pressure or you could injure the ear canal.

*Available in the United States and in Canada.

Check the solution as it drains into the emesis basin. Look for wax and excess medication. Then, check the ear with an otoscope, following the procedure outlined in the NURSING PHOTOBOOK *Assessing Your Patients*. If the ear canal still appears impacted, discard the drainage and repeat the procedure.

**3** When you've removed all the softened wax and excess medication from the patient's ear, wash the skin around the ear with soap and water. Avoid leaving any medication or wax on her skin. Then, instruct her to lie on her affected side for several minutes to make sure complete drainage has occurred. Clean and dry the outer ear canal to prevent skin excoriation.

## Administering ear drops

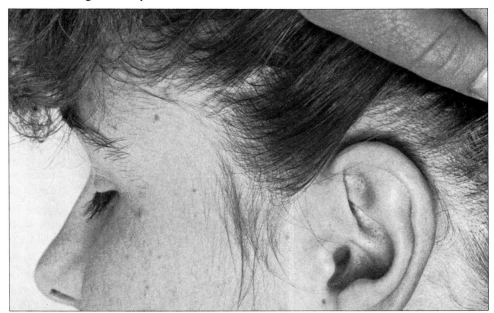

**1** *Imagine that you work in a large clinic and the first patient you see one morning has a painful ear infection. To treat the condition, the doctor orders neomycin sulfate (Otobiotic) ear drops. Do you know how to administer them? This photostory will show you.*

Begin the procedure by washing your hands, and checking the medication label against the doctor's order. Warm the solution to body temperature by holding the bottle between your hands for 2 minutes. Never administer ear drops that aren't body temperature, because this could cause vertigo.

Explain the procedure to your patient. Then, place her on her side, so the affected ear is accessible.

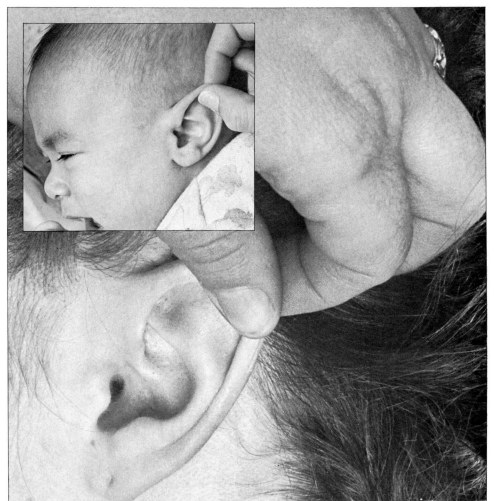

**2** Straighten the ear canal by gently pulling the auricle *up and back*. Remember, an infected ear is usually very painful. Be gentle.

[Inset] If your patient's a child, pull the auricle *down and back*.

# Ear medications

### Administering ear drops continued

**3** Taking care not to touch the ear with the dropper, instill the prescribed number of drops. Direct them along the side of the canal. By doing so, you avoid trapping any air in the ear. Then, hold the ear, as the nurse is doing here, until the medication disappears down the canal. Your patient will be able to tell you when the drops reach her tympanic membrane.

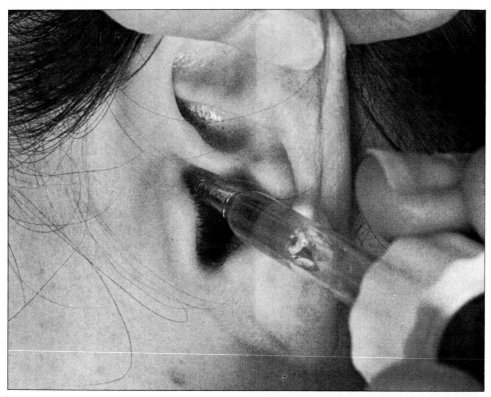

**4** Instruct your patient to remain on her side for about 10 minutes to keep the medication in the canal. Placing a medication-soaked cotton plug in her ear will also help. But don't use a dry cotton plug; it may absorb the medication.

Do both of the patient's ears require medication? Let her stay on her side for 10 minutes, then repeat the procedure in her other ear.

Finally, document the procedure, as well as your observations, in your nurses' notes.

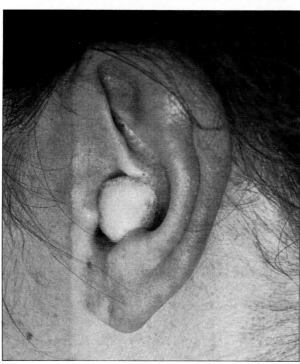

PATIENT TEACHING

**Teaching your patient to use ear drops**

Will your patient be using ear drops when he goes home? Make sure he knows how to administer them properly before he leaves the hospital. Review the steps for giving ear drops shown on pages 141 and 142. Let him do the procedure himself while you explain it to him in terms he can understand. Answer his questions. Finally, give him a completed copy of the home care aid on the next page.

# Patient teaching

# Home care

## Giving yourself ear drops

Dear Patient:

To relieve your ear infection, your doctor has prescribed these ear drops: _____
Use them exactly as directed on the label. Here's how:

• Begin by washing your hands thoroughly.

• Examine the medication. If it's discolored or has sediment in it, notify the doctor and get your prescription refilled. If nothing's wrong with the medication, proceed to the next step.

• For your own comfort, warm the medication by holding the bottle between your hands for 2 minutes.

• Shake the bottle, if directed, and open it.

• Fill the dropper; then, place the open bottle and dropper within easy reach.

• Lie on your side so the ear you're treating is exposed.

• Gently pull the top of your ear up and back, to straighten the ear canal.

• Position the dropper above your ear, taking care not to touch your ear with it. Squeeze the dropper's bulb to release one drop.

• Wait until you feel the drop in your ear. Then, if directed, squeeze the bulb again. Repeat this step until you've administered the prescribed number of drops.

• To keep the drops in your ear, continue to lie on your side for about 10 minutes.

• If you wish, plug your ear with cotton moistened with ear drops. Don't plug your ear with dry cotton, unless the doctor directs. Dry cotton will absorb the drops.

• If the doctor directs, repeat the procedure for the other ear.

• Recap the bottle. Store your drops away from light and extreme heat.

Important: Call your doctor immediately if you have any of these side effects: _____
_____
_____

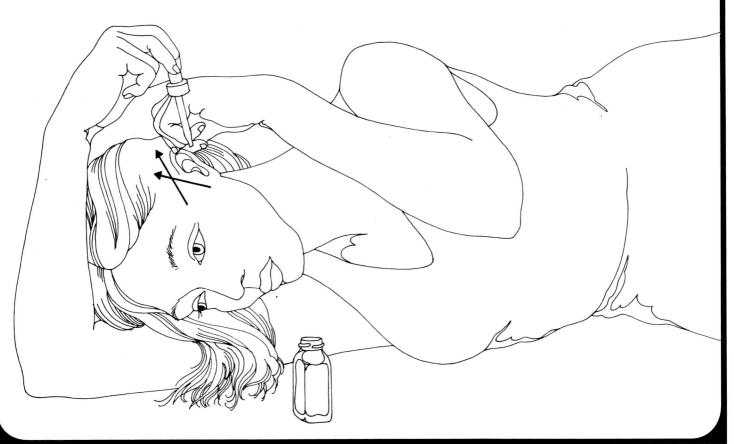

# Mouth and throat medications

The oral medications you give your patient aren't all intended for systemic absorption. Some, like pharyngeal sprays, mouthwashes, and lozenges (troches), are used for their local action on the patient's mouth and throat. Which one the doctor prescribes will depend, of course, on your patient's condition.

For example, if your patient has a local infection of the mouth or throat, the doctor may want you to administer an antibiotic mouth gargle, such as nystatin (Mycostatin*). To relieve postop throat soreness from an endotracheal tube, the doctor may want you to use an anesthetic spray containing lidocaine hydrochloride (Xylocaine*).

Learn about the various oral mucosal medications available by referring to the *Nurse's Guide to Drugs*. To find out how to administer oral mucosal medications—and teach your patient home care— read the following pages.

*Available in the United States and in Canada.

**Examining your patient's mouth and throat**

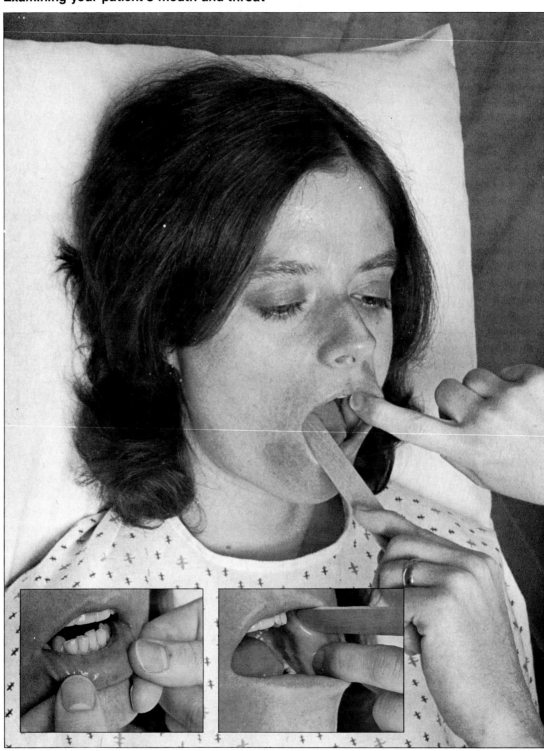

Before you administer any mouthwash or gargle, examine your patient's mouth and throat. Begin by using a tongue depressor to check her tongue, throat, and tonsils. Look for inflammation, ulcers, or white pustules, and document your observations.

Then, examine the insides of her lips and cheeks, as the nurse is doing in the inset photos. Check for inflammation, ulcers, and white pustules. Then, record your observations as before. By taking these notes, you can document your patient's progress—or lack of it—during treatment.

## Spraying your patient's mouth or throat

**1** *Does your patient have a sore throat? To relieve her pain and promote healing, the doctor may want you to spray it with a local antiseptic or anesthetic. Here's how, using an atomizer or spray pump:*

First, gather this equipment: an atomizer or spray pump containing the ordered medication, a spoon, and tissues. Make sure the medication's warmed to 100° F. (37.8° C.) by setting its container in warm water. However, take care not to wet the spray nozzle.

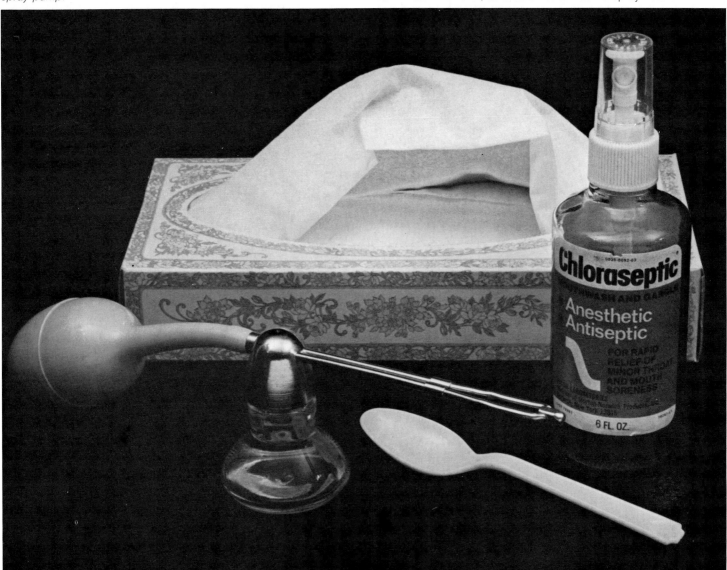

**2** Seat your patient upright, and explain the procedure to her. *Important:* If the patient can't sit up, ask the doctor if he can substitute another form of medication. Spraying the throat of a supine patient increases the risk of aspiration.

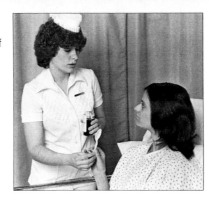

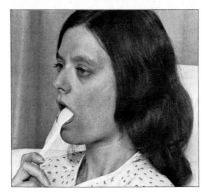

**3** Ask the patient to open her mouth. If you're administering an anesthetic, such as Chloraseptic, invert the bowl of a teaspoon over the patient's tongue *before* you spray. Ask her to hold it. This will keep her tongue from getting numb. It will also help you see the irritated area of her throat. Instruct the patient to avoid inhaling as the medication's being administered.

# Mouth and throat medications

### Spraying your patient's mouth or throat continued

**4** Are you using a spray pump? Hold the nozzle just *outside* the patient's mouth, and direct the medication toward her throat.

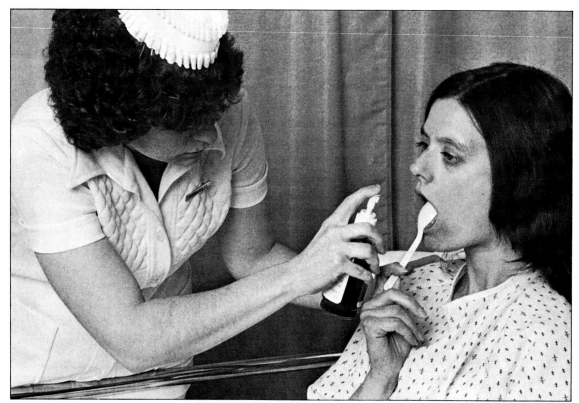

**5** If you're using an atomizer, insert its tip just *inside* the patient's mouth, and direct the medication toward the back of her throat.

Squeeze the container quickly and firmly, using enough force to propel the spray to the inflamed throat tissues. Caution the patient not to swallow immediately, so the medication can run down her throat and coat the mucous membranes. Stay alert, in case she aspirates the medication.

*Important:* If you've administered an anesthetic spray, warn your patient not to eat or drink anything for at least 1 hour afterward. The anesthetic will inhibit her gag reflex and increase the risk of aspiration.

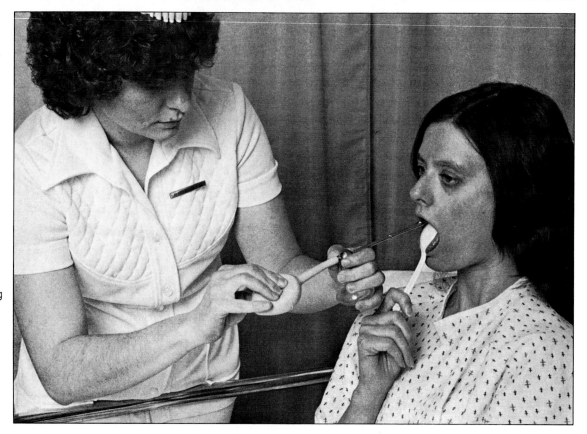

## How to administer a mouthwash or gargle

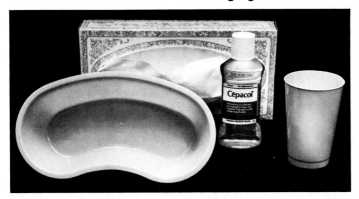

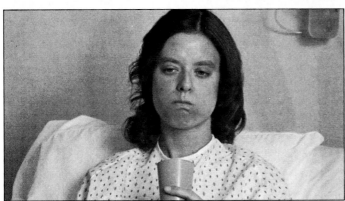

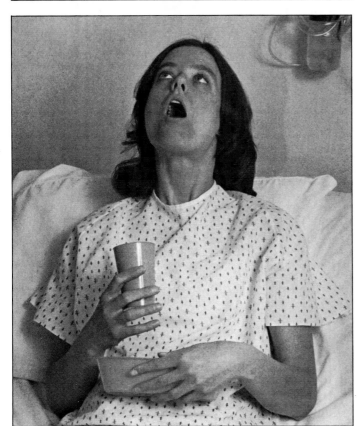

**1** *Suppose the doctor orders a mouthwash or gargle for your patient. Follow this administration procedure:*

Gather the solution, a drinking cup, an emesis basin, and tissues. Warm the solution by immersing its container in hot water. The container should be warm to your touch.

**2** Does the doctor want your patient to use the solution as a mouthwash? Then, seat your patient upright or ask her to stand, if she's able. Instruct her to swish ⅛ to ½ cup (30 to 59 ml) of the solution around in her mouth, especially over her teeth and gums. Warn her not to swallow it. Instead, instruct her to spit it into the emesis basin. Hand her a tissue so she can wipe her mouth.

**3** What if the doctor wants your patient to gargle with the solution? Seat her upright, with her head erect or tilted back slightly. Warm the solution, as explained earlier. Ask the patient to take a deep breath. Then, give her ⅛ cup of the solution, and tell her to hold it in her mouth. Then, instruct her to exhale slowly, to create the gargling action. But warn her not to aspirate the solution. Tell her to spit the solution into the emesis basin. Then, give her a tissue to wipe her mouth.

*Important:* If the doctor's ordered a medication like lidocaine hydrochloride (Xylocaine Viscous*), he may want you to instruct the patient to *swallow* the solution, so it coats and soothes irritated throat tissue. Tell her not to eat or drink for a half hour afterward.

Finally, document the procedure in your nurses' notes.

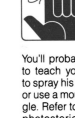

SPECIAL CONSIDERATIONS

**Administering lozenges**

If you're administering a lozenge (troche), instruct the patient not to chew it. Instead, tell him to keep it in his mouth until it dissolves.

*Caution:* Some lozenges contain sugar. If your patient's on a sugar-restricted diet, consult the doctor for a substitute medication.

PATIENT TEACHING

**Teaching mouth and throat home care**

You'll probably find it easy to teach your patient how to spray his mouth or throat or use a mouthwash or gargle. Refer to the preceding photostories for step-by-step instructions. Then, emphasize the following points:
• Place the spray or mouthwash bottle in warm water before use.
• Sit upright or stand during the administration procedure to avoid gagging.
• Don't eat for at least 30 minutes afterwards. If the spray has an anesthetic effect, don't eat for at least 1 hour afterwards. Otherwise, you may have trouble swallowing.

# Vaginal medications

Does administering vaginal medication to your patient make you uncomfortable? That's a normal reaction: you probably dislike embarrassing your patient and causing her pain. But you can minimize both of these concerns by learning how to do the procedures skillfully.

Read the following pages for special hints on how to irrigate your patient's vagina and administer medication. Within this section, you'll also find a handy home care aid you can copy for your patient.

### Performing a vaginal irrigation

**1** *You'll perform a vaginal irrigation on a female patient to prepare her for vaginal surgery, treat a vaginal infection, or reduce copious discharge. Here's how to do it:*
Begin the procedure by gathering the following irrigation equipment: a bag or bulb with tubing, an emesis basin, bedsaver pads, bedpan, water-soluble jelly, towel, sterile gloves, cotton balls; not shown, Betadine solution or soap and water, and an I.V. pole.

Before entering the patient's room, fill the douche bag with the prescribed solution.

Examine the tubing and nozzle that's attached to the bulb or bag. The special nozzle will have holes along its sides, rather than on the end, to minimize the chance of introducing irrigating solution into the patient's uterus.

Provide absolute privacy for your patient. Schedule the irrigations at times other than visiting hours, so you won't have to ask visitors to leave.

Ask your patient to empty her bladder. A distended bladder will cause unnecessary discomfort during the procedure.

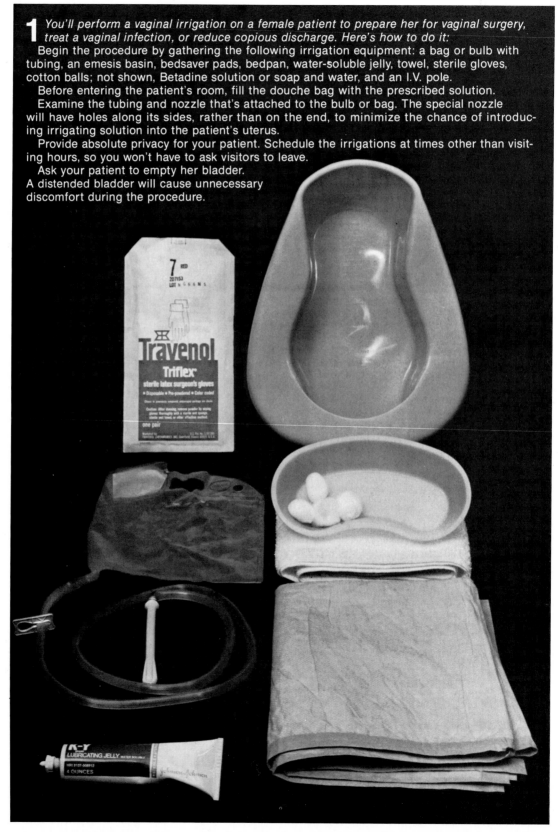

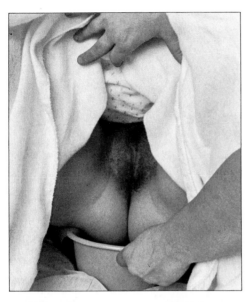

**2** Have your patient lie down with her buttocks on a bedpan, her knees flexed, and her legs spread apart. Place a drape over her legs, leaving only her perineum exposed. Raise the head of the bed about 30°. Place bedsaver pads under the patient.

Slip on a pair of sterile gloves and observe clean technique throughout the entire procedure.

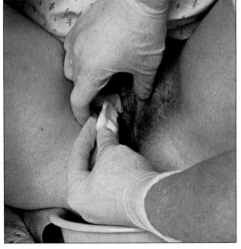

**3** Use cotton balls soaked in soapy warm water to clean the patient's perineum of any discharge. Work from the outer edges of the perineum inward.

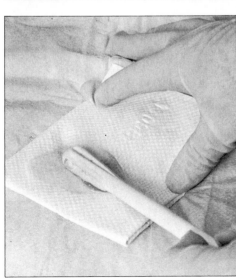

**4** Lubricate the nozzle with water-soluble jelly. Make sure the solution's body temperature or a little warmer. Then, hang the douche bag 12" (30.5 cm) above the vagina, on an I.V. pole. Flush the tubing with the solution. Close the roller clamp.

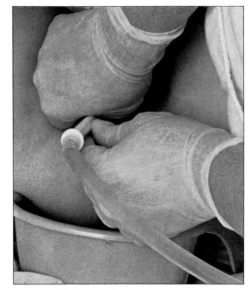

**5** With one hand, spread apart the patient's labia. Gently insert the nozzle into her vagina and angle it slightly up, then down toward her sacrum. Advance the nozzle tip about 2" (5 cm) into the vagina to ensure adequate irrigation.

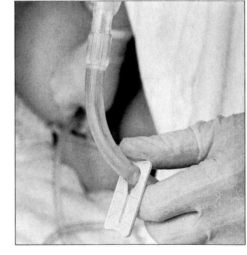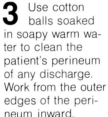

**6** Open the clamp on the tubing, and let gravity draw the solution into the vagina. Slowly rotate the nozzle, advancing it 1" to 2" (2.5 to 5 cm) as you do. But never rotate the nozzle if the patient has cervical cancer, or if she's had recent vaginal surgery.

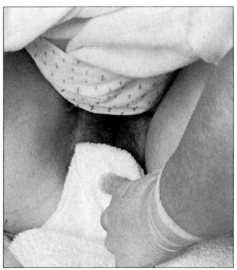

**7** When you've administered all the solution, remove the nozzle and bedpan. Use a towel to pat dry the patient's perineum and buttocks. Document the procedure. Finally, clean the equipment with soap and hot water, so it's ready for future use.

# Vaginal medications

### Administering a vaginal medication

**1** *Consider this possibility: One of your female patients has severe vaginitis and the doctor orders vaginal medication for her. You'll administer it using almost the same procedure we just described for irrigation. However, some differences exist. Read this photostory to learn what they are.*

First, gather the equipment: the prescribed medication (suppository, cream, ointment, tablet, or gel), applicator, sterile gloves, water-soluble gel, a paper towel, bedpan, bedsaver pad, several cotton balls, perineal pads, drape, and soap and water. Then, provide for the patient's privacy, and explain the procedure to her. Ask her to empty her bladder.

Have her lie down, with her knees flexed and legs spread apart. Place a bedsaver pad under the patient to protect the bed linen, and a drape over her legs, leaving only her perineum exposed.

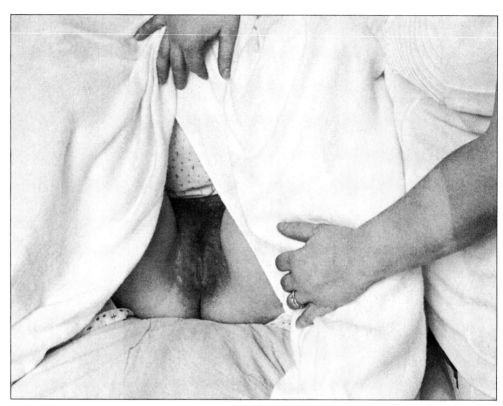

**2** Put on sterile gloves, and examine her perineum. If you see any discharge, you should wash the area. To do this, soak several cotton balls in soapy warm water. Then, clean the left side of the perineum, the right side, and finally the center, using a fresh cotton ball for each stroke.

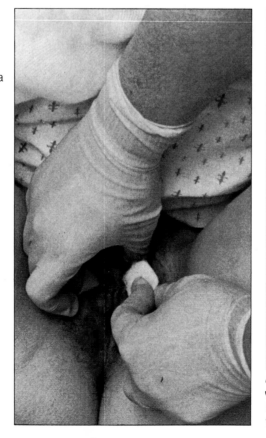

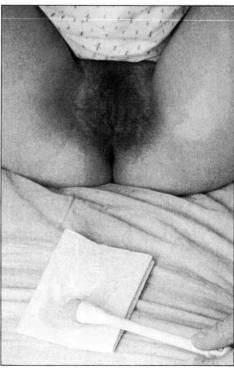

**3** Then, insert the prescribed dose of medication in the applicator. Next, lubricate the applicator tip with water or water-soluble gel, to make insertion easier.

**4** With one hand, spread apart the patient's labia. Gently insert the applicator into her vagina. Advance the applicator about 2" (5 cm), angling it slightly toward her sacrum. Then, push the plunger to instill the gel, ointment, or cream, or to release the tablet or suppository, as shown in the inset.

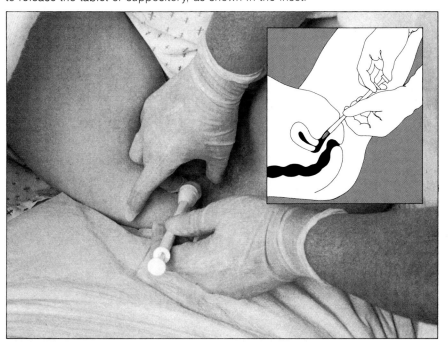

**5** Remove the applicator and discard it, if it's disposable. If it's reusable, wash it well with warm water and soap, and return it to its container.

Tell the patient to remain lying down for about 30 minutes. If she doesn't, the medication will run out, because the vagina has no sphincter. Apply perineal pads so her clothes or the bed linen don't become stained.

*Important:* Watch her closely for possible side effects, such as increased irritation, that may be caused by the medication. Notify the doctor if any occur.

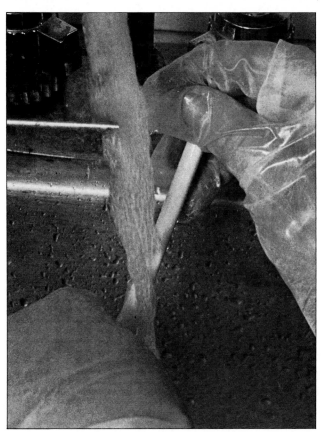

# Appendices

## Nurse's guide to dosage calculations

### LIQUID MEASURE EQUIVALENTS

| Apothecary | Approximate metric equivalent |
|---|---|
| 1 gallon | 3,800 milliliters |
| 1 quart | 950 milliliters |
| 1 pint | 475 milliliters |
| 8 fl. ounces (½ pint) | 240 milliliters |
| 4 fl. ounces | 120 milliliters |
| 2 fl. ounces | 60 milliliters |
| 1 fl. ounce | 30 milliliters |
| 15 minims | 1 milliliter |
| 10 minims | 0.6 milliliter |

### SOLID MEASURE EQUIVALENTS

| Apothecary | Approximate metric equivalent |
|---|---|
| 1 ounce | 30 grams |
| 15 grains | 1 gram |
| 10 grains | 600 milligrams |
| 7½ grains | 500 milligrams |
| 5 grains | 300 milligrams |
| 1½ grains | 100 milligrams |
| 1 grain | 60 milligrams |
| ¾ grain | 50 milligrams |
| ½ grain | 30 milligrams |
| ⅜ grain | 25 milligrams |
| ¼ grain | 15 milligrams |
| ⅙ grain | 10 milligrams |
| ⅛ grain | 8 milligrams |
| 1/10 grain | 6 milligrams |
| 1/12 grain | 5 milligrams |
| 1/20 grain | 3 milligrams |
| 1/30 grain | 2 milligrams |
| 1/60 grain | 1 milligram |
| 1/100 grain | 600 micrograms |
| 1/150 grain | 400 micrograms |
| 1/200 grain | 300 micrograms |
| 1/250 grain | 250 micrograms |
| 1/300 grain | 200 micrograms |

### METRIC EQUIVALENTS

| 1 kilogram | 1000 liters |
|---|---|
| 1 decaliter | 10 liters |
| 1 liter | 1000 milliliters |
| 1 milliliter | 1000 microliters |
| 1 kilogram | 1000 grams |
| 1 decagram | 10 grams |
| 1 gram | 1000 milligrams |
| 1 milligram | 1000 micrograms |

### INFUSION RATE EQUIVALENTS

| 1 milliliter | 60 microdrops |
|---|---|
| 1 milliliter | 15 drops |
| 1 drop | 4 microdrops |
| 1 drop | 1 minim |

If you work in a large hospital, the pharmacy probably supplies most medications prepackaged and ready to administer. Doing so obviously makes your work easier, but what happens when you must calculate dosage yourself? Will you know how? To help you, we've assembled an approximate equivalent table on the left. Review it. Then, see how these equivalents are used in the common calculation problems that follow.

*Conversion within the same system of measure*

• The doctor orders 0.75 gm of tetracycline hydrochloride. The tetracycline hydrochloride you have on hand is in milligrams. How many milligrams should you administer to fill the doctor's order?
   First, set up a proportion equal to one, using, as your numerator, the system of measure of the drug on hand (milligrams) and, as your denominator, the system of measure of the ordered drug (grams). Multiply this equation by the ordered amount (0.75 gm):

$$0.75 \text{ gm} \times \frac{1000 \text{ mg}}{1 \text{ gm}} = X$$

$$750 \text{ mg} = X$$

• Suppose the tetracycline is in 250-mg capsules. How many capsules would you give to fill the doctor's order? Divide the ordered amount by the capsule amount:

$$\frac{750 \text{ mg}}{250 \text{ mg}} = X$$

$$3 = X$$

• The doctor orders 600 mcg of vitamin $B_{12}$. The vitamin $B_{12}$ on hand is in milligrams. How many micrograms should you administer to fill the doctor's order? Set up a proportion equal to one, using, as your numerator, the system of measure of the drug on hand (mg) and, as your denominator, the system of measure of the ordered drug (mcg). Multiply this equation by the ordered amount (600 mcg):

$$600 \text{ mcg} \times \frac{1 \text{ mg}}{1000 \text{ mcg}} = X$$

$$\frac{600 \text{ mg}}{1000} = X$$

$$0.6 \text{ mg} = X$$

*Conversion from one system of measure to another*

• The doctor orders 1/200 grain of atropine sulfate. The atropine on hand is in milligrams. How many milligrams would you administer to fill the doctor's order?
   Set up a proportion equal to one, using, as your numerator, the system of measure of the drug on hand (mg) and, as your denominator, the system of measure of the ordered drug (grain). Multiply this equation by the ordered amount (1/200 grain):

$$\frac{1}{200} \text{ grain} \times \frac{60 \text{ mg}}{1 \text{ grain}} = X$$

$$\frac{60 \text{ mg}}{200} = X$$

$$0.3 \text{ mg} = X$$

• The doctor orders 600 mg of aspirin. The aspirin on hand is in

5-grain tablets. How many tablets should you administer to fill the doctor's order?

Set up a proportion equal to one, using, as your numerator, the system of measure of the drug on hand (grain) and, as your denominator, the system of measure of the ordered drug (mg). Multiply this equation by the ordered amount (600 mg):

$$600 \text{ mg} \times \frac{1 \text{ grain}}{60 \text{ mg}} = X$$

$$\frac{600 \text{ grains}}{60} = X$$

$$10 \text{ grains} = X$$

Then, divide 10 grains by the number of grains in each tablet:

$$\frac{10 \text{ grains}}{5 \text{ grains}} = X$$

$$2 = X$$

• The doctor orders 0.6 mg scopolamine. The scopolamine on hand is in grains. How many grains would you administer to fill the doctor's order?

Set up a proportion equal to one, using as your numerator the system of measure of the drug on hand (grain) and, as your denominator, the system of measure of the ordered drug. Multiply this equation by the ordered amount (0.6 mg):

$$0.6 \text{ mg} \times \frac{1 \text{ grain}}{60 \text{ mg}} = X$$

$$\frac{0.6 \text{ grain}}{60} = X$$

$$\frac{1}{100} \text{ grains} = X$$

*Determining infusion rates*

• The doctor orders 1000 ml of 10% dextrose in water to be given over 4 hours. How do you determine the per-minute rate?

Set up this equivalent: Place the ordered amount over the ordered time and the unknown amount over 1 minute.

$$\frac{1000 \text{ ml}}{240 \text{ mins}} = \frac{X \text{ ml}}{1 \text{ min}}$$

$$1000 \text{ ml/min} = 240 \, X$$

$$4 \text{ ml/min} = X$$

Then read the packaging information on the I.V. set you're using to find out how many drops per milliliter the set delivers. Suppose it delivers 15 drops per ml. To deliver 4 mls per minute, you'd have to multiply 15 by 4, to get the flow rate of 60 drops per minute.

• The doctor orders 0.25 mg/kg of amphotericin B to be given daily in 1000 ml of 5% dextrose in water over 6 hours. How do you determine the per-minute infusion rate?

First, you learn that your patient weighs 154 lbs. To convert his weight into kilograms, you multiply it by a proportion of one, with 1 kg as your numerator and its equivalent, 2.2 pounds, as your denominator.

$$154 \text{ lbs} \times \frac{1 \text{ kg}}{2.2 \text{ lbs}} = X$$

$$70 \text{ kg} = X$$

Then multiply his weight in kilograms (70 kg) by the ordered amount (0.25 mg/kg):

$$70 \text{ kg} \times \frac{0.25 \text{ mg}}{1 \text{ kg}} = X$$

$$17.5 \text{ mg} = X$$

Add 17.5 mg of amphotericin B to the 1000 ml of 5% dextrose in water. To determine the infusion rate, multiply your I.V. set's drip rate (15 gtts) by the ordered amount of I.V. fluid (1000 ml) over the ordered time in minutes (360 mins).

$$\frac{15 \text{ gtts}}{1 \text{ min}} \times \frac{1000 \text{ ml}}{360 \text{ mins}} = X$$

$$\frac{15000 \text{ gtts}}{360 \text{ mins}} = X$$

$$41 \text{ gtts/min} = X$$

*Determining reconstitution percentages*

• The doctor orders 300,000 units of penicillin G sodium I.M. The vial on hand contains 1,000,000 units of powdered penicillin. You know 2 ml is a safe amount of solution to administer I.M. You have to determine how much sterile saline solution must be added to the 1,000,000-unit penicillin vial so that you can draw out 2 ml and have it contain the ordered amount of penicillin. How do you do this?

Since you want to give 300,000 units in 2 ml, write this as a proportion and multiply it by the number of units in the vial:

$$\frac{2 \text{ ml}}{300,000 \text{ units}} \times 1,000,000 \text{ units} = X$$

$$\frac{2,000,000 \text{ ml}}{300,000} = X$$

$$6.6 \text{ ml} = X$$

• The doctor orders 2000 mg of sterile carbenicillin disodium (Geopen) in 5 ml of sterile water to be given I.V. The Geopen vial on hand contains 5 grams of powdered Geopen. You have to determine how much sterile water must be added to the 5-gram vial so that you can draw out 5 ml and have it contain the ordered amount of Geopen. How do you do this?

First, convert the system of measure on hand to the ordered system of measure:

$$5 \text{ grams} \times \frac{1000 \text{ mg}}{1 \text{ gram}} = X$$

$$5000 \text{ mg} = X$$

Then, multiply this figure by the amount of fluid ordered over the amount of drug ordered to get the amount of sterile water to add to the vial.

$$5000 \text{ mg} \times \frac{5 \text{ ml}}{2000 \text{ mg}} = X$$

$$\frac{25000 \text{ ml}}{2000} = X$$

$$12.5 \text{ ml} = X$$

For more information consult a standard reference on dosage calculations.

# Appendices

## I.V. compatibility chart: solutions and medications

This chart details the compatibility and incompatibility of drugs with I.V. solutions.

A drug is considered compatible with I.V. solution or another medication if, when mixed with either, it doesn't lose its potency or cause a significant loss of potency in the other medication.

Incompatibility occurs when a drug mixed with an I.V. solution or another drug is consequently rendered unsuitable for administration—either because it becomes toxic, or because it undergoes some physical change, such as precipitation.

If the drug you want to add to I.V. solution isn't listed here, don't assume it's either compatible or incompatible. Instead, call your hospital pharmacy for information.

Also, two drugs may be *physically* compatible, but not *therapeutically* compatible; in other words, the drugs when mixed might interact, altering the effect of one or both drugs. Read medication labels carefully. When in doubt, call your hospital pharmacy.

*Caution:* Avoid mixing multiple drugs in I.V. solutions whenever possible. The more drugs that are added, the greater the risk of incompatibility or interaction.

*Note: The amphotericin B row and column display the message "TO BE PREPARED BY PHARMACY" in place of compatibility data.*

| | albumin | amikacin | aminophylline | amino acid injection | amphotericin B | ampicillin | calcium gluconate | carbenicillin | cefamandole | cefazolin | cefoxitin | cephalothin | chloramphenicol | cimetidine | clindamycin | corticotropin (ACTH) | dexamethasone | dextrose 5% in water | dextrose 5% in lactated Ringer's | dextrose 5% in 0.45% NaCl | dextrose 5% in 0.9% NaCl | diazepam | diazoxide | diphenhydramine |
|---|---|---|---|---|---|---|---|---|---|---|---|---|---|---|---|---|---|---|---|---|---|---|---|---|
| albumin | X | O | O | O | | O | O | O | O | O | O | O | O | O | O | O | C | C | C | C | | ● | NR | O |
| amikacin | O | X | 8 | O | | ● | 24 | 8 | NR | 8 | NR | ● | 24 | 24 | 24 | O | ● | 24 | 24 | 24 | 24 | ● | NR | 24 |
| aminophylline | O | 8 | X | 24 | | O | C | O | O | O | O | ● | O | O | ● | ● | ● | C | C | C | C | ● | NR | C |
| amino acid injection | O | O | 24 | X | 12 | 24 | 24 | O | 24 | O | 24 | 1 | 24 | 24 | O | O | C | C | C | C | | ● | NR | C |
| amphotericin B | | | | | X | T | O | | B | E | | P | R | E | P | A | R | E | D | | B | Y | | P |
| ampicillin | O | ● | ● | ● | | X | ● | ● | ● | O | O | O | 1 | C | ● | O | O | 2 | 4 | 4 | 4 | ● | NR | O |
| calcium gluconate | O | 24 | C | 24 | | C | X | C | ● | ● | O | ● | C | O | ● | C | C | C | C | C | C | ● | NR | C |
| carbenicillin | O | 8 | C | 24 | | ● | C | X | O | C | O | O | O | O | ● | O | 24 | C | C | C | C | ● | NR | O |
| cefamandole | O | NR | O | O | | O | ● | O | X | O | O | O | O | O | O | O | O | C | C | C | C | ● | NR | O |
| cefazolin | O | 8 | O | 24 | | O | ● | C | O | X | O | O | 24 | 24 | O | O | O | C | C | C | C | ● | NR | O |
| cefoxitin | O | NR | O | O | | O | O | O | O | O | X | O | O | O | O | O | O | C | C | C | C | ● | NR | O |
| cephalothin | O | ● | ● | 24 | | ● | O | O | O | O | O | X | C | 24 | 24 | O | O | C | C | C | C | ● | NR | ● |
| chloramphenicol | O | 24 | O | T | 1 | C | ● | O | 24 | O | C | X | O | C | C | C | C | C | C | | ● | NR | C |
| cimetidine | O | 24 | O | O | | C | ● | O | 24 | O | 24 | O | X | 24 | 24 | O | O | C | C | C | C | ● | NR | O |
| clindamycin | O | 24 | ● | 24 | | O | O | 24 | O | O | O | 24 | O | 24 | X | O | O | C | C | C | C | ● | NR | O |
| corticotropin (ACTH) | O | O | ● | B | ● | C | O | O | O | O | O | O | C | O | O | X | O | C | C | C | C | ● | NR | O |
| dexamethasone | O | ● | ● | E | O | C | O | O | C | O | O | O | O | O | O | X | C | C | C | C | ● | NR | ● |
| dextrose 5% in water | C | 24 | C | C | 2 | C | C | C | C | C | C | C | C | C | C | C | C | X | O | O | O | ● | NR | C |
| dextrose 5% in lactated Ringer's | C | 24 | C | P | 4 | C | C | C | C | C | C | C | C | C | C | C | C | O | X | O | O | ● | NR | C |
| dextrose 5% in 0.45% NaCl | C | 24 | C | R | 4 | C | C | C | C | C | C | C | C | C | C | C | C | O | O | X | O | ● | NR | C |
| dextrose 5% in 0.9% NaCl | C | 24 | C | E | 4 | C | C | C | C | C | C | C | C | C | C | C | C | O | O | O | X | ● | NR | C |
| diazepam | ● | ● | ● | P | ● | ● | ● | ● | ● | ● | ● | ● | ● | ● | ● | ● | ● | ● | ● | ● | ● | X | ● | ● |
| diazoxide | NR | NR | NR | A | NR | NR | NR | NR | NR | NR | NR | NR | NR | NR | NR | NR | NR | NR | NR | NR | NR | ● | X | NR |
| diphenhydramine | O | 24 | C | R | O | C | O | O | O | O | O | ● | O | O | O | O | ● | C | C | C | C | ● | NR | X |
| dopamine | O | O | O | 24 | E | ● | 24 | 24 | O | O | O | 6 | 24 | O | O | ● | O | C | C | C | C | ● | NR | O |
| epinephrine | O | 24 | ● | O | D | O | ● | 24 | O | O | O | ● | ● | O | O | ● | O | C | C | C | C | ● | NR | O |
| erythromycin (I.V.) lactobionate | O | ● | C | 24 | | ● | C | O | ● | ● | O | ● | ● | NR | O | C | O | C | C | C | C | ● | NR | 24 |
| fat emulsion 10% & 20% | O | ● | ● | B | ● | O | ● | ● | ● | ● | ● | ● | ● | ● | ● | ● | ● | ● | ● | ● | ● | ● | ● | ● |
| gentamicin | O | NR | NR | Y | ● | NR | ● | NR | NR | NR | NR | ● | ● | 24 | 24 | O | O | C | C | C | C | ● | NR | NR |
| heparin sodium | O | ● | C | 24 | | ● | C | O | O | O | O | 8 | C | O | 24 | 24 | 4 | C | C | C | C | ● | NR | O |
| hydrocortisone Na succinate | O | O | C | P | C | C | C | 24 | O | O | O | 24 | C | O | 24 | 24 | 4 | C | C | C | C | ● | NR | ● |
| insulin (regular) | O | O | ● | H | O | O | O | O | O | O | O | 8 | O | 24 | O | O | O | C | C | C | C | ● | NR | O |
| isoproterenol | O | O | ● | A | O | O | C | O | O | O | O | O | O | O | O | O | O | C | C | C | C | ● | NR | O |
| kanamycin | O | O | C | R | ● | ● | ● | ● | O | O | 24 | O | ● | O | 24 | O | O | C | C | C | C | ● | NR | O |
| lactated Ringer's | C | O | C | M | 8 | C | C | C | C | C | C | C | C | C | C | C | NR | O | O | O | O | ● | NR | C |
| levarterenol | O | 24 | ● | A | O | O | C | O | O | O | O | ● | C | O | O | C | O | C | C | C | C | ● | NR | O |
| lidocaine | O | O | C | 24 | C | ● | C | C | C | O | O | O | C | O | O | O | C | C | C | C | ● | NR | C |
| metaraminol | O | 24 | O | 24 | Y | O | C | O | O | O | O | C | C | O | O | O | O | ● | C | C | C | ● | NR | ● |
| methicillin | O | ● | C | 24 | | O | C | O | O | O | O | ● | 1 | O | C | C | 6 | 6 | 6 | 6 | ● | NR | C |
| methylprednisolone | O | O | 6 | 24 | O | ● | ● | O | O | O | O | ● | C | O | 24 | O | O | C | C | C | C | ● | NR | O |
| miconazole | O | NR | NR | NR | N | NR | NR | NR | NR | NR | NR | NR | NR | NR | NR | NR | NR | C | NR | NR | NR | ● | NR | NR |
| multiple vitamin infusion (MVI) | O | O | O | C | L | O | C | O | O | C | 24 | O | O | O | 24 | O | O | C | C | C | C | ● | NR | O |
| nafcillin | O | O | 12 | O | Y | ● | O | O | O | O | O | O | C | O | O | O | C | C | C | C | ● | NR | C |
| nitroprusside | O | NR | NR | NR | | NR | NR | NR | NR | NR | NR | NR | NR | NR | NR | NR | C | NR | NR | NR | ● | NR | NR |
| 0.9% NSS | C | 24 | C | C | 8 | C | C | C | C | C | C | C | C | C | O | O | O | O | O | O | ● | NR | C |
| oxacillin | O | 8 | ● | 24 | | O | O | O | O | O | O | C | ● | O | O | C | C | C | C | C | ● | NR | O |
| oxytocin | O | O | O | O | | O | O | O | O | C | O | ● | O | O | O | C | C | C | C | C | ● | NR | O |
| penicillin G | O | 8 | ● | 24 | | O | C | O | O | C | O | O | C | 24 | 24 | C | C | C | C | C | ● | NR | C |
| phenytoin | ● | ● | ● | ● | | ● | ● | ● | ● | ● | ● | ● | ● | ● | ● | ● | ● | ● | ● | ● | ● | ● | | ● |
| phytonadione | O | 24 | ● | 24 | | O | O | O | O | O | O | O | C | O | O | C | C | C | C | C | ● | NR | C |
| polymyxin B | O | 24 | O | O | | ● | O | ● | O | ● | O | ● | O | O | O | O | C | NR | NR | NR | ● | NR | C |
| potassium chloride | O | 4 | C | 24 | | C | C | 24 | O | C | O | C | 24 | 24 | C | 4 | C | C | C | C | ● | NR | O |
| procainamide | O | NR | C | O | | O | C | O | O | O | O | O | C | O | O | O | O | O | O | ● | NR | C |
| sodium bicarbonate | O | 24 | C | O | | O | ● | 24 | O | 24 | C | C | C | 24 | O | O | C | C | C | C | ● | NR | O |
| tetracycline | O | 8 | ● | 24 | | O | ● | O | O | O | O | O | C | C | C | C | C | C | C | C | ● | NR | O |
| thiamine | O | ● | ● | O | | O | O | O | O | O | O | O | O | O | O | C | C | C | C | C | ● | NR | O |
| ticarcillin | O | ● | O | O | | ● | O | ● | O | ● | O | ● | O | O | O | O | O | C | C | C | C | ● | NR | O |
| tobramycin | O | O | O | O | | O | ● | ● | NR | ● | NR | ● | O | O | O | O | C | C | C | C | ● | NR | O |
| vancomycin | O | 24 | ● | O | | ● | O | O | O | ● | O | O | C | O | O | C | C | C | C | C | ● | NR | C |
| vitamin B complex with C | O | 24 | ● | O | | C | ● | O | C | 24 | C | ● | 24 | 24 | C | 4 | C | C | C | C | ● | NR | C |

**Key:**    C = Compatible    ● = Incompatible    NR = Not recommended by the manufacturer

| dopamine | epinephrine | erythromycin lactobionate | fat emulsion 10% & 20% | gentamicin | heparin sodium | hydrocortisone Na succinate | insulin (regular) | isoproterenol | kanamycin | lactated Ringer's | levarterenol | lidocaine | metaraminol | methicillin | methylprednisolone | miconazole | multiple vitamin infusion (MVI) | nafcillin | nitroprusside | 0.9% NSS | oxacillin | oxytocin | penicillin G | phenytoin | phytonadione | polymyxin B | potassium chloride | procainamide | sodium bicarbonate | tetracycline | thiamine | ticarcillin | tobramycin | vancomycin | vitamin B complex with C |
|---|---|---|---|---|---|---|---|---|---|---|---|---|---|---|---|---|---|---|---|---|---|---|---|---|---|---|---|---|---|---|---|---|---|---|---|
| ○ | ○ | ○ | ○ | ○ | ○ | ○ | ○ | ○ | ○ | C | ○ | ○ | ○ | ○ | ○ | ○ | ○ | ○ | ○ | C | ○ | ○ | ○ | ● | ○ | ○ | ○ | ○ | ○ | ○ | ○ | ○ | ○ | ○ | ○ |
| ● | 24 | ● | ● | ○ | ● | ○ | ○ | ○ | ○ | ○ | 24 | ○ | 24 | ● | ○ | NR | ○ | ○ | NR | 24 | 8 | ○ | 8 | ● | 24 | 24 | 4 | NR | ○ | 8 | ○ | ● | ○ | 24 | 24 |
| ○ | ● | C | ● | NR | C | C | ● | ● | C | C | ● | C | ○ | C | 6 | NR | ○ | 12 | NR | C | ● | ○ | ● | ● | ● | ○ | C | C | C | ● | ○ | ○ | ○ | ● | ● |
| 24 | ○ | 24 | ● | 24 | 24 | ○ | 24 | 24 | C | C | 24 | 24 | 24 | 24 | 24 | NR | C | ○ | NR | C | 24 | ○ | 24 | ● | 24 | ○ | 24 | ○ | ○ | 24 | ○ | ○ | ○ | ○ | ○ |
| **H** | **A** | **R** | **M** | **A** | **C** | **Y** | | **O** | **N** | **L** | **Y** | | | | | | | | | | | | | | | | | | | | | | | | |
| ● | ○ | ● | ● | ● | ● | C | ○ | ○ | ● | 8 | ○ | ● | ● | ● | ○ | NR | ○ | ● | NR | 8 | ● | ○ | ● | ● | ● | ● | C | ○ | ○ | ● | ○ | ● | ○ | ○ | ● |
| 24 | ● | C | ● | NR | C | C | ○ | C | ● | C | C | C | ○ | C | ● | NR | C | ○ | NR | C | ○ | ○ | C | ● | ○ | ○ | C | C | ● | ● | ○ | ○ | ● | C | C |
| 24 | ● | ● | ● | ● | ○ | 24 | ○ | ○ | ● | C | ○ | C | ○ | ○ | ○ | NR | ○ | ○ | NR | C | ○ | ○ | ○ | ● | ○ | ● | 24 | ○ | 24 | ● | ○ | ○ | ● | ○ | ● |
| ○ | ○ | ○ | ● | NR | ○ | ○ | ○ | ○ | ○ | C | ○ | C | ○ | ○ | ○ | NR | ○ | ○ | NR | C | ○ | ○ | ○ | ● | ○ | ○ | ○ | ○ | ○ | ○ | ○ | ○ | NR | ○ | ○ |
| ○ | ○ | ● | ● | NR | ○ | ○ | ○ | ○ | ● | C | ○ | ○ | ○ | ○ | ○ | NR | C | ○ | NR | C | C | C | C | ● | ○ | ● | C | ○ | ○ | ● | ○ | ○ | ● | ○ | C |
| ○ | ○ | ○ | ● | NR | ○ | ○ | ○ | ○ | 24 | C | ○ | ○ | ○ | ○ | ○ | NR | 24 | ○ | NR | C | ○ | ○ | ○ | ● | ○ | ○ | ○ | ○ | 24 | ○ | ○ | ○ | NR | ○ | 24 |
| 6 | ● | ● | ● | ● | 8 | 24 | 8 | C | ● | C | ● | ● | C | ● | ● | NR | ○ | ○ | NR | C | ● | ○ | ● | ● | ● | ● | C | ○ | C | ● | ○ | ○ | ● | ○ | C |
| 24 | ○ | ● | ● | ● | C | C | ○ | ○ | C | C | ● | C | C | 1 | C | NR | ○ | C | NR | C | ● | C | C | ● | C | ● | C | C | C | ● | ○ | ○ | ○ | ● | ● |
| ○ | ○ | NR | ● | 24 | ○ | ○ | 24 | ○ | ○ | C | ○ | ○ | ○ | ○ | ○ | NR | ○ | ○ | NR | C | ○ | ○ | 24 | ● | ○ | ○ | 24 | ○ | C | ○ | ○ | ○ | ○ | ○ | 24 |
| ○ | ○ | ○ | ● | 24 | 24 | 24 | ○ | ○ | 24 | C | ○ | ○ | ○ | ○ | 24 | NR | 24 | ○ | NR | C | ○ | ○ | 24 | ● | ○ | ○ | 24 | ○ | 24 | ○ | ○ | ○ | ● | ○ | 24 |
| ○ | ○ | ○ | ● | NR | 24 | 24 | ○ | ○ | ○ | C | C | ○ | ○ | C | ○ | NR | ○ | ○ | NR | C | ○ | ○ | C | ● | ○ | ○ | C | ○ | ● | C | ○ | ○ | ○ | C | C |
| ○ | ○ | ○ | ● | NR | 4 | 4 | ○ | ○ | C | ○ | NR | C | ● | C | ○ | NR | ○ | C | NR | C | ○ | ○ | C | ● | C | ○ | 4 | ○ | ○ | C | ○ | ○ | ○ | ● | 4 |
| C | C | C | ● | C | C | C | ○ | C | C | ○ | C | C | C | 6 | C | C | C | C | NR | ○ | C | C | C | ● | C | C | C | C | C | C | C | C | C | C | C |
| C | C | C | ● | C | C | C | ○ | C | C | ○ | C | C | C | 6 | C | NR | C | C | NR | ○ | C | C | C | ● | C | NR | C | ○ | C | C | C | C | C | C | C |
| C | C | C | ● | C | C | C | ○ | C | C | ○ | C | C | C | 6 | C | NR | C | C | NR | ○ | C | C | C | ● | C | NR | C | ○ | C | C | C | C | C | C | C |
| C | C | C | ● | C | C | C | ○ | C | C | ○ | C | C | C | 6 | C | NR | C | C | NR | ○ | C | C | C | ● | C | NR | C | ○ | C | C | C | C | C | C | C |
| ● | ● | ● | ● | ● | ● | ● | ● | ● | ● | ● | ● | ● | ● | ● | ● | ● | ● | ● | ● | ● | ● | ● | ● | ● | ● | ● | ● | ● | ● | ● | ● | ● | ● | ● | ● |
| NR | NR | NR | ● | NR | NR | NR | NR | NR | NR | NR | NR | NR | NR | NR | NR | NR | NR | NR | NR | NR | NR | NR | NR | NR | NR | NR | NR | NR | NR | NR | NR | NR | NR | NR | NR |
| ○ | ○ | 24 | ● | NR | ○ | ● | ○ | ○ | ○ | C | ○ | C | ● | C | ● | NR | ○ | C | NR | C | ○ | ○ | C | ● | C | C | ○ | C | ○ | C | ○ | ○ | ○ | C | C |
| X | ○ | ○ | ● | 6 | 24 | ○ | ○ | ○ | 24 | C | ○ | 24 | ○ | ○ | 18 | NR | ○ | ○ | NR | C | 24 | ○ | 6 | ● | ○ | ○ | 24 | ○ | ● | 24 | ○ | ○ | ○ | ○ | ○ |
| ○ | X | ○ | ● | NR | ○ | ○ | ○ | ○ | ○ | C | ○ | 2 | C | ○ | ○ | NR | ○ | ○ | NR | C | ● | ○ | ● | ● | ● | ○ | ○ | ○ | ● | ● | ○ | ○ | ○ | ● | ● |
| ○ | ○ | X | ● | NR | ● | C | ○ | ○ | ○ | C | ○ | C | ● | C | ○ | NR | ● | ○ | NR | C | ○ | ○ | C | ● | ○ | C | C | ○ | 24 | ● | ● | ○ | ○ | ○ | ● |
| ● | ● | ● | X | ● | ● | ● | ● | ● | ● | ● | ● | ● | ● | ● | ● | ● | ● | ● | ● | ● | ● | ● | ● | ● | ● | ● | ● | ● | ● | ● | ● | ● | ● | ● | ● |
| 6 | NR | NR | ● | X | ● | NR | NR | NR | NR | C | NR | C | NR | NR | NR | NR | NR | ● | NR | C | ● | NR | NR | NR | NR | NR | NR | NR | NR | NR | NR | ● | NR | NR | ● |
| 24 | ● | ● | ● | ● | X | ● | ○ | 8 | ● | C | ● | 8 | ● | ● | C | NR | ○ | C | NR | C | ○ | ○ | ● | ● | ● | ● | C | C | ○ | ● | ○ | ○ | ● | ● | C |
| 18 | ○ | C | ● | NR | ● | X | 8 | ○ | ● | C | C | C | ● | ● | 4 | NR | ○ | ● | NR | C | ○ | ○ | C | ● | ○ | ○ | C | C | C | ● | ○ | ○ | ○ | ● | C |
| ○ | ○ | ○ | ● | NR | ○ | 8 | X | ○ | ○ | ○ | ○ | ● | ○ | ○ | ● | NR | ○ | ○ | NR | C | ○ | ○ | ● | ● | ○ | ○ | C | ● | ● | ○ | ○ | ○ | ○ | ○ | C |
| ○ | ○ | ○ | ● | NR | 8 | ○ | ○ | X | ○ | C | ○ | ● | ○ | ○ | ○ | NR | C | ○ | NR | C | ○ | ○ | ○ | ● | ○ | ○ | C | ○ | ● | C | ○ | ○ | ○ | ○ | C |
| 24 | ○ | ○ | ● | NR | ● | ● | ○ | ○ | X | C | ○ | ○ | C | ● | ○ | NR | ● | NR | NR | C | NR | ○ | C | ● | ○ | C | ○ | ○ | ○ | C | ● | ● | NR | NR | ● |
| C | C | C | ● | C | C | C | ○ | C | C | X | C | C | ● | 6 | C | NR | C | C | NR | ○ | C | C | C | ● | C | NR | C | ○ | C | C | C | C | C | C | C |
| ○ | ○ | ○ | ● | NR | ● | C | ○ | ○ | ○ | C | X | ● | ● | ● | C | NR | C | C | NR | NR | ● | ● | ● | ● | ○ | ○ | C | ○ | ● | ● | ○ | ○ | ○ | ○ | C |
| 24 | 2 | C | ● | C | 8 | C | ● | ● | | C | ● | X | C | ○ | ○ | NR | ○ | ○ | NR | C | ○ | ○ | C | ● | ○ | ○ | C | ○ | ● | C | ○ | ○ | ○ | ○ | C |
| ○ | C | ● | ● | NR | ● | ● | ○ | ○ | C | ● | ● | C | X | ● | ● | NR | ● | ● | NR | C | ● | C | ● | ● | ● | ○ | C | C | C | C | ○ | ○ | ○ | C | ● |
| ○ | ○ | C | ● | NR | ● | ● | ○ | ○ | ● | 6 | ● | ○ | ● | X | ○ | NR | ○ | ○ | NR | 6 | ○ | ○ | ● | ● | ● | C | C | NR | ● | ● | ○ | ○ | ○ | ● | ● |
| 18 | ○ | ○ | ● | NR | C | 4 | ● | ○ | ○ | C | C | ○ | ● | ○ | X | NR | ○ | ● | NR | C | ○ | ○ | ● | ● | ○ | ○ | C | ○ | C | ● | ○ | C | ○ | ○ | ● |
| NR | NR | NR | ● | NR | NR | NR | NR | NR | NR | NR | NR | NR | NR | NR | NR | X | NR | NR | NR | C | NR | NR | NR | ● | NR | NR | NR | NR | NR | NR | NR | NR | NR | NR | NR |
| ○ | ○ | ● | ● | NR | ○ | ○ | ○ | C | ● | C | C | ○ | ● | ○ | ○ | NR | X | ○ | NR | C | ○ | ○ | 4 | ● | ○ | ○ | C | ○ | ○ | ● | ○ | ○ | ○ | ○ | ○ |
| ○ | ○ | ○ | ● | ● | C | ● | ○ | ○ | ○ | C | C | ○ | ● | ○ | ● | NR | ○ | X | NR | C | ○ | ○ | ○ | ● | ○ | ○ | C | ○ | C | ● | ○ | ○ | ● | ○ | ● |
| NR | NR | NR | ● | NR | NR | NR | NR | NR | NR | NR | NR | NR | NR | NR | NR | NR | NR | NR | X | NR | NR | NR | NR | ● | NR | NR | NR | NR | NR | NR | NR | NR | NR | NR | NR |
| C | C | C | ● | C | C | C | C | C | C | ○ | NR | C | C | 6 | C | C | C | C | NR | X | C | C | C | ● | C | C | C | ○ | C | C | C | C | C | C | C |
| 24 | ● | ○ | ● | ● | ○ | ○ | ○ | ○ | NR | C | ● | ○ | ● | ○ | ○ | NR | ○ | ○ | NR | C | X | ○ | ● | ● | ● | ○ | C | ○ | ○ | ● | ○ | ○ | ○ | ○ | ● |
| ○ | ○ | ○ | ● | NR | ○ | ○ | ○ | ○ | ○ | C | ● | ○ | C | ○ | ○ | NR | ○ | ○ | NR | C | ○ | X | C | ● | C | ○ | ○ | ○ | ○ | C | ○ | ○ | ○ | ○ | ○ |
| 6 | ● | C | ● | NR | ● | C | ● | ○ | C | C | ● | C | ● | ● | ● | NR | 4 | ○ | NR | C | ● | C | X | ● | C | ● | C | C | ● | ● | ○ | ○ | ● | ● | ● |
| ● | ● | ● | ● | ● | ● | ● | ● | ● | ● | ● | ● | ● | ● | ● | ● | ● | ● | ● | ● | ● | ● | ● | ● | X | ● | ● | ● | ● | ● | ● | ● | ● | ● | ● | ● |
| ○ | ○ | ○ | ● | NR | ● | ○ | ○ | ○ | NR | C | ○ | ○ | ● | ● | | NR | ○ | ○ | NR | C | ● | C | C | ● | X | ○ | ○ | ○ | ○ | ○ | ○ | ○ | ○ | ● | ○ |
| ○ | ○ | C | ● | NR | ● | C | ○ | ○ | C | ○ | ○ | ○ | ○ | C | ○ | NR | ○ | ○ | NR | C | ○ | ○ | ● | ● | ○ | X | ○ | ○ | ○ | ● | ○ | ○ | ○ | ○ | C |
| 24 | ○ | C | ● | NR | C | C | C | C | ○ | C | C | C | C | C | C | NR | C | C | NR | C | C | ○ | C | ● | ○ | ○ | X | ○ | ○ | C | ○ | ○ | ○ | C | C |
| ○ | ○ | ○ | ● | NR | C | C | ● | ○ | ○ | ○ | ○ | ○ | C | NR | ○ | NR | ○ | ○ | NR | ○ | ○ | ○ | C | ● | ○ | ○ | ○ | X | ○ | C | ○ | ○ | ○ | C | C |
| ● | ● | 24 | ● | NR | ○ | C | ● | ● | ○ | C | ● | ● | C | ● | C | NR | ○ | C | NR | C | ○ | ○ | ● | ● | ○ | ○ | ○ | ○ | X | ● | ○ | ○ | ○ | ● | ● |
| 24 | ● | ● | ● | NR | ● | ● | ○ | C | C | ● | C | C | C | ● | ● | NR | ● | ● | NR | C | ● | C | ● | ● | ○ | ● | C | ○ | ● | X | ○ | ○ | ○ | ○ | ● |
| ○ | ○ | ● | ● | NR | ○ | ○ | ○ | ○ | ● | C | ○ | ○ | ○ | ○ | ○ | NR | ○ | ○ | NR | C | ○ | ○ | ○ | ● | ○ | ○ | ○ | ○ | ○ | ○ | X | ○ | ○ | ○ | C |
| ○ | ○ | ○ | ● | ● | ○ | ○ | ○ | ○ | ● | C | ○ | ○ | ○ | ○ | C | NR | ○ | ○ | NR | C | ○ | ○ | ○ | ● | ○ | ○ | ○ | ○ | ○ | ○ | ○ | X | ● | ○ | ○ |
| ○ | ○ | ○ | ● | NR | ● | ○ | ○ | ○ | NR | C | ○ | ○ | ○ | ○ | ○ | NR | ○ | ● | NR | C | ○ | ○ | ● | ● | ○ | ○ | ○ | ○ | ○ | ○ | ○ | ● | X | ○ | ○ |
| ○ | ● | ○ | ● | NR | ● | ● | ○ | ○ | NR | C | ○ | ○ | C | ● | ○ | NR | ○ | ○ | NR | C | ○ | ○ | ● | ● | ● | ○ | C | C | ● | ○ | ○ | ○ | ○ | X | ● |
| ○ | ● | ● | ● | ● | C | C | C | C | ● | C | C | C | ● | ● | ● | NR | ○ | ● | NR | C | ● | ○ | ● | ● | ○ | C | C | C | ● | ● | C | ○ | ○ | ● | X |

○ = Data unavailable **2, 4, 8, 24** = Compatible only for the number of hours indicated **X** = Identical drug

# Acknowledgements

**We'd like to thank the following people and companies for their help with this PHOTOBOOK:**

ABBOTT LABORATORIES
North Chicago, Ill.

AMERICAN FOUNDATION FOR THE BLIND, INC.
New York, N.Y.
Alex H. Townsend

AUTO-SYRINGE, INC.
Hooksett, N.H.
William Arthur,
Vice President Marketing & Sales

BAXA CORPORATION
Northbrook, Ill.
Philip E. Smith,
Vice President Marketing

BITNER AND MCVAN PHARMACY
Lansdale, Pa.
John McVan, RPh

CARDIAC TREATMENT CENTERS, INC.
Camp Hill, Pa.

IVAC CORPORATION
San Diego, Calif.
Chérie M. Hawes, RN,
Clinical Specialist

JELCO LABORATORIES
Raritan, N.J.

MONOJECT
Division of Sherwood Medical
A Brunswick Company
St. Louis, Mo.
Aggie Sigsbee,
Professional Product Sales Representative

**Also the staffs of:**

DOYLESTOWN HOSPITAL
Doylestown, Pa.

MAGEE MEMORIAL HOSPITAL
Philadelphia, Pa.

TEMPLE UNIVERSITY HOSPITAL
Philadelphia, Pa.

THOMAS JEFFERSON UNIVERSITY HOSPITAL
Philadelphia, Pa.

# Selected references

**Books**

Ansel, Howard C. INTRODUCTION TO PHARMACEUTICAL DOSAGE FORMS, 2nd ed. Philadelphia: Lea & Febiger, 1976.

Barber, Janet M., et al. ADULT AND CHILD CARE: A CLIENT APPROACH TO NURSING. St. Louis: C.V. Mosby Co., 1977.

Belinkoff, Stanton. INTRODUCTION TO INHALATION THERAPY. Boston: Little, Brown & Co., 1969.

Bergersen, Betty S. PHARMACOLOGY IN NURSING, 14th ed. St. Louis: C.V. Mosby Co., 1979.

Bower, Fay Louise, and Em Olivia Bevis. FUNDAMENTALS OF NURSING PRACTICE: CONCEPTS, ROLES, AND FUNCTIONS. St. Louis: C.V. Mosby Co., 1979.

Dison, Norma. CLINICAL NURSING TECHNIQUES, 3rd ed. St. Louis: C.V. Mosby Co., 1975.

DuGas, Beverly W. KOZIER-DU GAS' INTRODUCTION TO PATIENT CARE, 2nd ed. Philadelphia: W.B. Saunders Co., 1972.

Egan, Donald F. FUNDAMENTALS OF RESPIRATORY THERAPY, 3rd ed. St. Louis: C.V. Mosby Co., 1977.

Falconer, Mary W., et al. THE DRUG, THE NURSE, THE PATIENT, 6th ed. Philadelphia: W.B. Saunders Co., 1978.

Fuerst, Elinor V., et al. FUNDAMENTALS OF NURSING: THE HUMANITIES AND THE SCIENCES IN NURSING, 5th ed. Philadelphia: J.B. Lippincott Co., 1974.

Goldstein, Avram, et al. PRINCIPLES OF DRUG ACTION: THE BASIS OF PHARMACOLOGY, 2nd ed. New York: John Wiley & Sons, Inc., 1974.

Goodman, L.S., and A. Gilman. THE PHARMACOLOGICAL BASIS OF THERAPEUTICS, 5th ed. New York: Macmillan Co., 1975.

Harmer, Bertha. TEXTBOOK OF THE PRINCIPLES AND PRACTICE OF NURSING, 5th ed. New York: Macmillan Co., 1955.

Johns, Marjorie P. DRUG THERAPY AND NURSING CARE. New York: Macmillan Co., 1979.

Kozier, Barbara, and Glenora Lea Erb. FUNDAMENTALS OF NURSING: CONCEPTS AND PROCEDURES. Reading, Mass.: Addison-Wesley Pub. Co., 1979.

LaDu, Bert N., et al. FUNDAMENTALS OF DRUG METABOLISM AND DISPOSITION. Baltimore: Williams & Wilkins Co., 1971.

Levine, Ruth R. PHARMACOLOGY: DRUG ACTIONS AND REACTIONS. Boston: Little, Brown & Co., 1973.

MANAGING I.V. THERAPY. Nursing80® Photobook™ Series. Horsham, Pa.: Intermed Communications, Inc., 1980.

Martin, Eric, et al. TECHNIQUES OF MEDICATION: A MANUAL OF THE ADMINISTRATION OF DRUG PRODUCTS. Philadelphia: J.B. Lippincott Co., 1969.

Modell, Walter, et al. APPLIED PHARMACOLOGY. Philadelphia: W.B. Saunders Co., 1976.

NEEDLE AND CANNULA TECHNIQUES. North Chicago: Abbott Laboratories, 1971.

NURSE'S RESPONSIBILITY IN I.V. THERAPY, THE. North Chicago: Abbott Laboratories, 1972.

PARENTERAL ADMINISTRATION. North Chicago: Abbott Laboratories, 1970.

Phipps, W.J., et al. MEDICAL SURGICAL NURSING. St. Louis: C.V. Mosby Co., 1979.

Plumer, A.L. PRINCIPLES AND PRACTICES OF INTRAVENOUS THERAPY. Boston: Little, Brown & Co., 1970.

PROVIDING RESPIRATORY CARE. Nursing80® Photobook™ Series. Horsham, Pa.: Intermed Communications, Inc., 1979.

Rodman, Morton J., and Dorothy W. Smith. PHARMACOLOGY AND DRUG THERAPY IN NURSING. Philadelphia: J.B. Lippincott Co., 1968.

Saunders, W., and R. Gardier. PHARMACOTHERAPY IN OTOLARYNGOLOGY. St. Louis: C.V. Mosby Co., 1976.

Sorensen, Karen C., and Joan Luckmann. BASIC NURSING. Philadelphia: W.B. Saunders Co., 1979.

Strauss, Steven. PATIENT DOSAGE INSTRUCTIONS. Ambler, Pa.: Medical Business Service, 1976.

**Periodicals**

Black, C.D., et al. *Drug Interactions in the GI Tract,* AMERICAN JOURNAL OF NURSING. 77:1426-1429, September 1977.

Boyles, V.A. *Injection Aids for Blind Diabetic Patients,* AMERICAN JOURNAL OF NURSING. 77:1456-1458, September 1977.

Brandt, P.A., et al. *I.M. Injections in Children,* AMERICAN JOURNAL OF NURSING. 72:1402-1406, August 1972.

Burke, E.L. *Insulin Injection: The Site and the Technique,* AMERICAN JOURNAL OF NURSING. 72:2194-2196, December 1972.

Chezem, J.L. *Locating the Best Thigh Injection Site,* NURSING73. 3:20-21, December 1973.

Croft, C.L. *BCG Administration and Nursing Implications,* AMERICAN JOURNAL OF NURSING. 77:315-319, February 1979.

Dodd, M.J. *Theoretical Bases of Immunotherapy,* AMERICAN JOURNAL OF NURSING. 77:310-314, February 1979.

Engle, V. *Diabetic Teaching,* NURSING75. 5:17-24, December 1975.

Fischer, A. *(Insulin) Injection Site Selection Made Simple,* PATIENT CARE. 12:185, February 15, 1978.

Geolot, D.H., and N.P. McKinney. *Administering Parenteral Drugs,* AMERICAN JOURNAL OF NURSING. 75:788-793, May 1975.

Greenblatt, David J., and Jan Kock-Weser. *Intramuscular Injection of Drugs,* NEW ENGLAND JOURNAL OF MEDICINE. 295:542-546, September 2, 1976.

Hays, D. *Do It Yourself the Z-track Way,* AMERICAN JOURNAL OF NURSING. 74:1070-1071, June 1974.

Hussar, Daniel A. *Drug Interactions: Good and Bad,* NURSING76. 6:61-65. January 1976.

Kelleher A., et al. *Drug Therapy by Indwelling Arterial Catheter,* AMERICAN JOURNAL OF NURSING. 75:1990-1992, November 1975.

Knowles, J.A. *The Art of Intramuscular Injection,* DRUG THERAPY. 5:149-47, November 1975.

Kurdi, W.J. *Refining Your I.V. Therapy Techniques,* NURSING75. 5:41-47, November 1975.

Lambert, Martin L. *Drug and Diet Interactions,* AMERICAN JOURNAL OF NURSING. 75:402-406, March 1975.

Lang, S.H., et al. *Reducing Discomfort from I.M. Injections,* AMERICAN JOURNAL OF NURSING. 76:800-801, May 1976.

Lowenthal, Werner. *Factors Affecting Drug Absorption,* AMERICAN JOURNAL OF NURSING. 73:1391-1408. August 1973.

Newton, D.W., and M. Newton. *Needles, Syringes and Sites for Injectable Medications,* JOURNAL OF AMERICAN PHARMACY ASSOCIATION. 17:685-687, November 1977.

Nysather, J., et al. *The Immune System—Its Development and Functions,* NURSING76. 6:1614-1616, October 1976.

Pitel, M. *The Subcutaneous Injection,* AMERICAN JOURNAL OF NURSING. 71:76-79, January 1971.

Pitel, M., and M. Wemmett. *The Intramuscular Injection,* AMERICAN JOURNAL OF NURSING. 64:104-109, April 1964.

# Index

## A

Absorption of drugs, 15
  dermatomucosal, 120
  gastrointestinal, 20-21
  parenteral, 64, 71, 78-79, 84-85
  respiratory, 100-101, 108-109
Acetylcysteine, 110-111
Additive set infusion. See
  *Intermittent I.V. infusion.*
Aerosol therapy drugs, 110-111
AFB needle guide, 76
Alcoholic solution, 25. See also
  *Oral medications.*
Allergy, drug, 13
Antecubital fossa, anatomy, 85
Atelectasis, 116
Atomizer
  home care aid, 106
  patient teaching, 105
Atrophy, skin, 74
Auto-Syringe Syringe Pump®
  See *Infusion pressure
  equipment.*

## B

Bacille Calmette-Guerin. See
  *BCG.*
Basilic veins, location of, 84-85
Bath. See *Medicated bath.*
Baxa Bottle Adaptor and Dis-
  pensor, using a, 29
BCG, 68. See also *Immunother-
  apy.*
  administering with Heaf gun, 69
Beclomethasone dipropionate,
  110-111
Biotransformation of drugs, 15
Body medications, applying,
  126-127. See also *Skin
  medications.*
Bolus injection. See *Direct bolus
  method.*
Bronkometer. See *Metered-dose
  nebulizer.*
Buccal route, 35

## C

Capsules. See *Oral medications,
  tablets and capsules.*
Cephalic veins, location of, 84-
  85
Circulatory depression, 116
Compatibility chart, I.V. solutions
  and medications, 154-155
Continuous drip method
  advantages/disadvantages, 85
  how to use, 90-91
  using a vented bottle or a
    bag, 92
*Corynebacterium Parvulum.* See
  *C Parvum.*
C Parvum, 68. See also *Immunotherapy.*
Cream, skin, 121. See also *Skin
  medications.*

Cromolyn sodium, 110-111

## D

Debriding agent, applying, 128
Deltoid site (injection), 79
Dexamethasone sodium phos-
  phate, 110-111
Diabetic patient
  injection equipment for visually
    impaired, 76-77
  teaching self-injection, 74-75
Diagnostic skin test
  antigens, 65
  reading, 68
Direct bolus method
  advantages/disadvantages, 85
  how to use, 88-89
Distribution of drugs, 15
Documenting, 16-17
Dorsogluteal site (injection), 79
Dosage calculation, nurse's
  guide to, 152-153
Dos-Aid Syringe Filling Device, 76
Douche, administering a. See
  *Vaginal medications, irriga-
  tion.*
Dressing. See *Medicated dress-
  ing, applying.*
Drip method. See *Continuous
  drip method.*
Drug absorption. See *Absorption
  of drugs.*

## E

Ear irrigation. See *Ear medications, irrigation.*
Ear medications
  drops, administering, 141-142
  home care aid (administering
    ear drops), 142-143
  irrigation, 140-141
Effervescent tablets, 25. See
  also *Oral medications.*
Elderly patient and medications,
  16, 35. See also *Diabetic
  patient, injection equipment
  for visually impaired; Identa-
  Drug Wallet®; Medication
  clocks.*
Elixir (type of alcoholic solution),
  25. See also *Oral medications.*
Emulsion (type of suspension),
  25. See also *Oral medications.*
Epinephrine 1:1,000, 110-111
Excretion of drugs, 15
Eye irrigation. See *Eye medications, irrigation.*
Eye medications
  drops, instilling, 134-135
  home care aid (administering
    eye drops), 139
  irrigation, 132-133
  ointment, instilling, 136-137
  patch, applying, 138

Eye patch. See *Eye medications,
  patch, applying.*

## F

Facial medications, applying,
  124-125
Five Rights system, 8-10
Fluidextract (type of alcoholic
  solution), 25. See also *Oral
  medications.*
Foley catheter, 36. See also
  *Gastrostomy tube.*

## G

Gargle. See *Mouth and throat
  medications.*
Gastrointestinal absorption. See
  *Absorption of drugs, gas-
  trointestinal.*
Gastrostomy dressing. See
  *Gastrostomy tube, changing
  dressing.*
Gastrostomy tube
  changing dressing, 48
  home care aid (caring for
    gastrostomy), 49
  how to unclog, 47
  patient teaching, 48
  types, 36
Gel (type of suspension), 25.
  See also *Oral medications.*

## H

Heaf gun, 69. See also *Immunotherapy.*
Heparin, injecting, 74
Histoplasmin, 65. See also
  *Diagnostic skin test.*
Home care aids
  atomizer, how to use, 106
  ear drops, self-administration,
    143
  eye drops, self-administration,
    139
  gastrostomy care, 49
  insulin injection, self-adminis-
    tration, 75
  medicated cream or ointment,
    how to apply, 129
  metered-dose nebulizer, 114
  nasal aerosol device (Turbi-
    naire®), how to use, 107
  oral medications, general
    guidelines, 33
  sitz bath, how to take, 131
  turbo-inhaler, how to use, 112-
    113
Hyperglycemia, 74
Hypertrophy, skin, 74
Hypoglycemia, 74

## I

Identa-Drug Wallet®, 32
Immunotherapy, 68-69

advantages/disadvantages, 68
Heaf gun, using, 69
Infiltration. See *Intravenous administration, complications.*
Infusion pressure equipment
  Auto-Syringe Syringe Pump®, 95
  infusion pump, 95
  pressure bag, 95
Infusion pump. See *Infusion pressure equipment.*
Inhalation therapy
  advantages/disadvantages, 108
  aerosol therapy drugs, 110-111
  home care aids
    metered-dose nebulizer, how to use, 114
    turbo-inhaler, how to use, 112-113
  how it works, 108-109
  IPPB therapy, 116
  oxygen delivery system, 117
  oxygen therapy complications, 116
  patient teaching, 111
  vaporizer, 115
Injection sites
  intradermal, 64
  intramuscular, 78-79
  intravenous, 84-85
  subcutaneous, 70
Injection tips, 63
Instillation, nasal
  characteristics of medications, 102
  home care aids
    atomizer, how to use, 106
    nasal aerosol device (Turbinaire®), how to use, 107
  nose drops, administering
    adult, 103-104
    infant/child, 105
  patient teaching, 105
  positioning patient for sinus treatment, 102
  upper airway anatomy, 100-101
Insulin injection
  home care aid (self-injection), 75
  mixing two types, 74
  patient teaching, 74
Intermittent I.V. infusion
  advantages/disadvantages, •85
Intra-arterial administration
  changing a dressing, 96-97
  complications, 97
  infusion equipment, 95
  managing an arterial line, 96
  preparing patient, 96
Intradermal administration. See also *Immunotherapy.*
  diagnostic skin antigens, 65
  injecting medication, 66-67
  injection sites, 64

reading diagnostic skin tests, 68
Intramuscular administration
  complications, 83
  injecting medication, 80-82
  injection sites, 78-79
  pros and cons, 78
  Z-track method, 83
Intravenous administration
  administration methods
    advantages/disadvantages of each, 85
    continuous drip, 90-91
    direct bolus, 88-89
    intermittent infusion, 85
    intermittent infusion, 85
    piggyback I.V., 93
    secondary I.V., 93
  bag, using a, 92
  choosing venipuncture site, 84-85
  indications/contraindications, 84
  medication hints, 93
  pediatric patient, 93
  performing venipuncture, 86-87
  vented bottle, using a, 92
IPPB therapy, 116
Isoetharine, 110-111
Isoproterenol hydrochloride, 110-111
I.V. bolus. See *Direct bolus method.*
I.V. compatibility chart: solutions and medications, 154-155
I.V. push. See *Direct bolus method.*

**L**

Legal responsibility, 14
Levin® tube, 36. See also *Nasogastric tube.*
Liquid medications. See *Oral medications.*
Lilly needle guide, 77
Lotion, skin, 121. See also *Skin medications.*
Lozenges, administering, 147

**M**

Magma (type of suspension), 25. See also *Oral medications.*
Mantoux, 65. See also *Diagnostic skin test.*
Medicated bath
  administering, 130
  sitz bath, 131
Medicated cream or ointment. See *Home care aids, medication cream or ointment, applying; Skin medications.*
Medicated dressing, applying, 130
Medication cart, 10
Medication clocks, 34

Medication, knowing the, 10
Medication syringe, 27-29
Medications, pre-pouring, 11
MER (methanol extract residue), 68. See also *Immunotherapy.*
Metaproterenol sulfate, 110-111
Metered-dose nebulizer
  home care aid (how to use), 114
  using a, 110
Methanol extract residue. See *MER.*
Monoject scale magnifier, 77
Mouth and throat, examining, 144. See also *Mouth and throat medications.*
Mouth and throat medications
  how to administer
    gargle, 147
    lozenges, 147
    mouthwash, 147
    spray, 145-146
Mouthwash. See *Mouth and throat medications.*
Mushroom catheter, 36. See also *Gastrostomy tube.*

**N**

Nasal aerosol device (Turbinaire®). See *Home care aids, nasal aerosol device (Turbinaire®), how to use; Turbinaire Decadron Phosphate.*
Nasal cannula, 117
Nasal catheter, 117
Nasogastric tube
  insertion, 37-41
  removal, 44
  types, 36
  using to give medication, 42-43
  special considerations, 44
Needles, 63
Nitroglycerin ointment, applying, 127. See also *Skin medications.*
Nonretention enema. See also *Rectal medications.*
  administering, 54-55
  withdrawing, 56
NPH insulin (drawing up with regular insulin), 74

**O**

Ointment, skin, 121, See also *Skin medications.*
Old tuberculin, 65. See also *Diagnostic skin test.*
Oral medications
  absorption, 20-21
  administering to child, 31
  administering to patient with tracheostomy, 31
  administering to stroke victim, 31

# Index

advantages/disadvantages, 22
liquids, 25
  administering to infant, 30-31
  administering with medication syringe, 27
  administering unpalatable medications, 29
  administering using Baxa Bottle Adaptor and Dispensor, 29
  patient teaching and home care aid, 32-35
  systemic (sublingual or buccal routes), 35
  tablets and capsules, 22-23
    administering, 23-24
    how they differ, 22
    mixing with food or beverage, 22-23
    storing, 23
Oxygen therapy
  complications, 116
  delivery systems, 117
Oxygen toxicity, 116

## P

Parenteral absorption. See *Absorption of drugs.*
Parkinson position, 102
Paste, skin, 121. See also *Skin medications.*
Pediatric patients
  administering nose drops to infant, 105
  administering oral medications to child, 31
  administering oral medications to infant, 30-31
  performing venipuncture on infant, 85
  preparing child for injection, 63
  special considerations during I.V. therapy, 93
Piggyback I.V. set, understanding and using, 93
Powder, reconstituted. See also *Oral medications.*
  oral administration, 25
  parenteral administration, 62
Powder, skin, 121. See also *Skin medications.*
Pressure bag. See *Infusion pressure equipment.*
Proetz position, 102

## R

Reconstituted powder. See *Powder, reconstituted.*
Rectal medications
  nonretention enema, 50-5l
    administering, 54-55
    withdrawing, 56
  ointment, 50
    applying, 58-59
  pros and cons, 50

retention enema, 50-51
    administering, 52-53
    retaining, 54
  suppository, 50
    inserting, 57-58
Rectal ointments. See *Rectal medications, ointment.*
Rectus femoris site (injection), 79
Respiratory depression, 116
Respiratory tract anatomy, 100-101
Retention enema. See also *Rectal medications.*
  administering, 52-53
  learning about, 50-51
  preparing to administer, 51
  retaining, 54

## S

Salem sump® tube, 36. See also *Nasogastric tube.*
Scalp medication, applying, 122-123. See also *Skin medications.*
Secondary I.V. set, understanding and using, 93
Simple face mask, 117
Sitz bath, administering, 130-131
Skin medications
  body medication, applying, 126-127
  debriding agent, applying, 128
  facial medication, applying, 124-125
  home care aids
    medicated cream or ointment, how to apply, 129
    sitz bath, how to take, 132
  medicated bath, administering, 131
  medication dressing, applying, 130
  nitroglycerin ointment, applying, 127
  nurse's reaction to skin conditions, 122
  pros and cons, 121
  scalp medication, applying, 122-123
  topical dosage forms, 121
Skin preps, 63
Skin test. See *Diagnostic skin test.*
Speed shock. See *Intravenous administration, complications.*
Spinhaler® See *Turbo-inhaler.*
Spirits (type of alcoholic solution), 25. See also *Oral medications.*
Spraying mouth or throat. See *Mouth and throat medications.*
Subcutaneous administration
  home care aid (insulin injection, self-administration), 75

injecting heparin, 74
  injecting medication, 72-73
  injection sites, 70-71
  special equipment for visually impaired diabetic, 76-77
  teaching diabetic, 74
  when to use, 70
Sublingual route, 35
Suppository, rectal. See *Rectal medications, suppository.*
Suspension, 25. See also *Oral medications.*
Syringe
  injection, 62
  medication, 27-29
Syringe pump. See *Infusion pressure equipment.*
Syrup, 25. See also *Oral medications, tablets and capsules.*
Systemic infection. See *Intravenous administration, complications.*

## T

Tablet. See *Oral medications, tablets and capsules.*
Thrombophlebitis. See *Intravenous administration, complications.*
Tincture (type of alcoholic solution), 25. See also *Oral medications.*
Topical dosage forms, 121. See also *Skin medications.*
Tuberculin purified protein derivative, 65. See also *Diagnostic skin test.*
Turbinaire Decadron Phosphate, 110
  home care aid (how to use), 107
  patient teaching, 105
Turbo-inhaler (Spinhaler®), 110
  home care aid (how to use), 112-113
  patient teaching, 111
Tyloxapol, 110-111

## V

Vaginal irrigation. See *Vaginal medications, irrigation.*
Vaginal medications
  administering, 150-151
  irrigation, 148-149
  patient teaching, 151
  preventing complications, 151
Vaporizer, 115. See also *Inhalation therapy.*
Venipuncture, 86-87
  site selection, 84-85
Ventrogluteal site (injection), 78
Vastus lateralis site (injection), 79

## Z

Z-track injection method, 83